Survival Guide for Nursing Students

Survival Guide for Nursing Students

Philip Burnard
PhD, MSc, RMN, RGN, DipN, CertEd, RNT

*Director of Postgraduate Nursing Studies, University of Wales
College of Medicine, Cardiff*

and

Paul Morrison
PhD, BA, RMN, RGN, PGCE, CPsychol, AFBPsS

*Lecturer in Nursing Studies, University of Wales College of
Medicine, Cardiff*

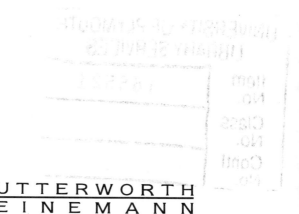

BUTTERWORTH
HEINEMANN

Butterworth-Heinemann Ltd
Linacre House, Jordan Hill, Oxford OX2 8DP

A member of the Reed Elsevier group

OXFORD   LONDON   BOSTON
MUNICH   NEW DELHI   SINGAPORE   SYDNEY
TOKYO   TORONTO   WELLINGTON

First published 1993

British Library Cataloguing in Publication Data
Burnard, Philip
   Survival Guide for Nursing Students
   I. Title   II. Morrison, Paul
   610.73

ISBN 0 7506 1589 3

Composition by TecSet Ltd, Wallington, Surrey
Printed and bound in Great Britain by Biddles Ltd, Guildford and King's Lynn

Contents

Preface

Whom is this book for?

Surviving as a nursing student can be a tough business. Some people sail through it. More find they have to work at producing essays, listening to lectures, developing interpersonal, clinical and computing skills. The book is for anyone who needs instant ideas and support during their time as a student nurse. It is mostly for students on nursing diploma and undergraduate courses but we hope it will also be useful to postgraduate and mature students. Returning to learning can also be fraught.

What is in the book?

The book is practical. Its chapters offer clear information about studying and working. It is divided up into a series of chapters that can be read straight through or on their own. The chapters include details about:

- Planning your work
- Organizing time
- Working with tutors and lecturers
- Using the library
- Keeping references
- Writing essays and projects
- Doing research
- Using computers
- Being assertive

- Communicating with others
- Preparing a CV
- Being interviewed

All in all, we hope that the chapters cover the sorts of problems that you are likely to encounter on a nursing course whether that course is located in a college, a school or a university and how to solve them.

How can I use the book?

You can read the book straight through if you want. You are more likely to want to pick out particular chapters as they become appropriate. We would advise you to treat this as a book to be *used*. Write in the margins, underline the things that you think are important, turn over the corners of the pages if you need to. This is not a textbook, nor a formal reference book. It is designed to be practical and useful.

Philip Burnard and Paul Morrison

Acknowledgements

This book has grown out of our experiences as both students and lecturers. Until recently, we were both. However, some of the best advice for the book has come from students on the courses we teach. Thanks to all the students who have talked to us in the course of our writing this book. Particular thanks to: Lisa Jenking, Tina Ann Bubear, Neil Simon Russel, and Karen Rendle and to all the other students who made such important contributions to the preparation of this book. Thanks, also, to the Terence Higgins Trust and the Family Planning Association for supplying a considerable amount of useful information.

Acknowledgements are given to Barclays Bank Ltd for permission to reproduce their students' financial checklist, to the Royal College of Nursing for permission to reproduce their Nursing Students' Bill of Rights and to the UKCC for permission to reprint their Guide for students of nursing and midwifery.

1

Being a student

Aims of the chapter

- To explore the best and worst things about being a nursing student.
- To identify ways of coping with the academic and practical aspects of being a nursing student.

Students' views of being a student

You are a student again. You have become a nursing student or you are looking forward to being one. What is it going to be like? In preparing this book, we asked a number of student nurses about the process of being a student. In this chapter, we explore some of their reactions, and consider the implications of their ideas for you. In the chapters that follow, we offer practical suggestions about how to survive. First, though, the students speak.

What are the good and bad things about being a nursing student? Nursing is both rewarding and exciting. It can also be hard work. Being a student and studying nursing can be particularly difficult. You have to combine both the academic with the practical. Sometimes the mix works: sometimes it does not. On the other hand, you have to *make* it work to survive. And this is what this book is all about.

Best things about being a student

The students that we talked to identified a range of issues that they considered were the 'best' things about being a student of nursing. Here are some of the things that they talked about:

- Lack of 'real life' responsibilities
- The complete contrast to the restrictions of earlier school experience
- Social life
- Status
- Reductions with student union cards
- Independence
- Making new friends
- Freedom

Many also liked being away from home, being their own boss and being able to do what they liked, when they liked. Others liked the new style of learning and appreciated being able to work at their own pace and learning more about nursing skills and about themselves.

Worst things about being a student

They also discussed some of the worst things about student life. In deciding how to survive, it is important to know what you are letting yourself in for. These are some of the issues that our students mentioned:

- Stress related to work
- Essay deadlines
- Lack of confidence
- Lack of funds
- Group gossip
- Leaving parents, old friends and girlfriends
- Living, breathing, eating and working with friends

A number of students found that the organization of time, having to get down to hard work and a certain lack of will power were sometimes a problem, as was the question of combining work and social life.

Coping with practical and academic work

Nursing offers an interesting mix of practical work with people, alongside the academic study of a number of subjects. You somehow have to try to marry the two. This is what the students we talked to had to say about combining theory and practice:

- Practical work allows you to put theory into real life situations.
- Experiencing real life situations is helpful.
- In the practical setting, there is not always enough encouragement from lecturers.
- It is sometimes difficult to meet deadlines for academic work.
- People in practical settings do not always know what we are supposed to do.
- Sometimes the teachers are out of touch with the practical setting.

Most students thought that it was quite difficult to mix the academic side of courses with the practical side and some felt that there was an element of cramming involved in getting through all of the academic work that was involved in the various courses of study.

Mixing with other sorts of students

Nursing students are hybrids. While they are students in the sense of being attached to a college or a university, they are also 'working', too. In some ways, nursing education follows an apprenticeship format. You spend some of your time in college studying the theory of nursing. You spend a great deal of time working in clinical placements learning to be a nurse. These are some comments from the students that we talked to:

- If you apply yourself as expected, the course is far more intense than an 'ordinary' one. But, then again, you get a good all-round view of the practical and academic aspects of nursing.

- Some 'other' students do not appreciate the amount of work we have to do for the academic side of the course.
- Some people do not think that nursing is an academic discipline.
- They sometimes lack an understanding of the demands that patients make.
- There is sometimes animosity between the different sorts of nursing students on different courses.

Studying

Much of this book is about ways of organizing study. If there is one area that is likely to cause problems in nursing courses it is the need to balance working in clinical placements with academic work. It is also important to have enough free time to develop your social life. Sometimes, the juggling of those three things can cause problems. These are some of the points identified by our students:

- When deadlines are close, studying is very easy.
- It is very hard to study when you spend weekends at home with your boyfriend.
- It is difficult to study in a group of people. I find it easier to study on my own.
- Self-directed study requires discipline which is sometimes difficult to achieve.
- Inspiration is required from some lecturers in order to make studying easier.
- The most important parts of some subjects are left to us to find out on our own. This is not always easy.
- I would much rather socialize than work and there are plenty of opportunities to socialize.

Lecturers

Some lecturers are inspirational. Others are not. This is what the students we talked to had to say about lecturers and lectures:

- They should hand back work promptly.
- They should be willing to give extra tutorials.

- We should be allowed to evaluate the course more frequently.
- They should give lots of useful and relevant handouts.
- They should point out to students how to write essays before deadlines.
- They should make it blatantly obvious that lecturers are there to *help* and not just to teach and mark papers.
- They should show a friendly and non-judgemental attitude.

Clinical staff

Students work with trained nurses throughout their courses. Clinical staff are sometimes sympathetic to the needs of students and sometimes less so. This tension is illustrated by some of the students' comments:

- We should have more clinical experience.
- It should be made clear from the start if we have specific objectives to reach. These objectives should be made clear to ward staff, as well.
- Basic nursing skills should be taught *before* we get to work on the ward.
- Not all the clinical staff remember what it was like to be a student.
- The clinical nurses know what *real* nursing is like.
- The lecturers should spend more time working in the wards.
- We need to 'shadow' a qualified member of staff.

Useful resources

The list of possible resources for learning and studying is almost endless. These are some of the items that the students identified:

- The library – particularly periodicals
- The teaching staff
- Personal tutors
- The photocopier
- Wordprocessors
- Lecturers: when they help us to write essays
- Other people who have done the course

- The library is my second home
- CD-ROM
- Catalogues and bibliographies
- Other students – especially those who are on the same course but in a higher year
- Notice boards.

Students' advice to others

What would other students say to you as you start your course? Some might be less than encouraging as it is almost traditional to highlight the worst aspects of a new situation. But, some useful advice can be forthcoming. Here is what our students suggested:

- Try to find time to read the books on the reading lists.
- Get to know the library and how it works.
- Find time to relax and become involved in outside clubs and interests.
- Get to know wordprocessors.
- Don't get ill – it doesn't help.
- Learn to quote references properly.
- Try to keep a sense of balance between work and social life.
- Make use of the reading lists. Don't just put them in your folder and forget them.
- Don't rush out and buy lots of textbooks. Read around until you find one you really like.
- If you can't cope, find someone who will counsel you.
- Really enjoy the first few weeks. Don't be afraid to talk to people and have a chat.
- Keep a book-reference index.
- Work at developing a critical view of what you are taught in lectures.
- Enjoy yourself!

Coping with change

As you will gather from reading these comments, being a nursing student is a major life change. This book will help you to weather that change but most of the work has to be done by you, at your own pace and in your own individual way. What is most important is that you see all this as a *positive* life change. While all change can be destabling and disruptive, it can also be life enhancing and can lead to personal growth. *Notice* how you change over the next few months and years and notice how you cope with people, the job, the academic demands that are placed on you and the new skills that you learn as a result of all this. If you can, write down these reflections. In this way, you will be able to monitor the changes that take place.

Student checklist

The following are questions to reflect on when you consider becoming a student:

- What sort of student will I be?
- What are the things I am most and least looking forward to?
- How will I make new friends?
- What do I most want from this experience?

Summary of chapter

This chapter has offered a view of being a nursing student from the point of view of students, themselves. The aim has been to help you to identify various elements and issues in the process of becoming a nurse. The rest of the book is about managing the life change that comes about from being a nursing student.

2

Getting organized

Aims of the chapter

- To explore learning methods.
- To examine teaching methods used in nursing courses.
- To identify coping strategies.
- To enable planning.

Nursing is different to many types of study in that it combines two sorts of learning activity. On the one hand, there is practical, hands-on work in the clinical or community setting. On the other, there is academic study in the college. The former is usually structured in such a way as to enable you to learn as you work. Most clinical areas have well-defined learning objectives and most senior staff are trained to help you to make best use of your time. This chapter describes and discusses some of the factors that you need to bear in mind when getting organized with your studies. It discusses both the clinical and the academic aspects of nursing training and education.

What do I have to do?

The first part of any learning programme involves planning. You need to know the following things:

- What has to be learned.
- What learning facilities have been organized.
- How learning will be demonstrated.

This short-list of three elements covers almost the whole of the formal learning experience. First, you need to know what is *required learning*. In other words, what sorts of things do you need to know in order to become a nurse? Those 'things' are often divided into three:

- Nursing knowledge
- Nursing skills
- Nursing attitudes

These are self-explanatory. Nursing has its own body of knowledge and it also draws on other disciplines: anatomy and physiology, the behavioural sciences, medicine, pharmacology and so on. You need to know, right at the beginning of your course, the outline for learning these facets of nursing. On most courses, students are given a handbook that outlines the course in some detail. If you do not get such a handbook, ask to see the syllabus of training. Every college of nursing is required to draw up such a syllabus and it contains an outline of the knowledge and skills that will be taught in a nursing course.

There are numerous skills to be learned during a nursing course. A short list of these would include the following:

- Interpersonal skills
- Practical nursing skills
- Management skills
- Skills in coping with feelings
- Social skills

The line between knowledge and skills is sometimes a fine one. 'Knowledge' is usually thought of as something that can be written down in books and papers. 'Skills' are usually thought of as involving behaviour. On the other hand, the two sometimes shade into one another. If you are listening to another person, for example, you may be looking at them and nodding your head but you may also be drawing on knowledge from psychology and counselling theory.

Attitudes refer to the way we feel about things – the characteristic ways that we respond to people and situations. In the past, it was often thought that you could teach the 'right' attitudes towards certain nursing situations. Increasingly, though, it is realized that people react to various situations in different ways. What is important is that we learn to *notice* how we feel in various nursing encounters and learn to monitor the way we treat others and ourselves.

Knowledge, skills and attitudes are interlinked. Nursing is made up of 'facts' that have to be learned, behavioural and social skills that are used in all aspects of nursing care and of our personal attitudes towards patients and colleagues. Most modern approaches to learning in colleges of nursing offer challenging and imaginative ways of learning nursing. Most, too, acknowledge that it is important to bridge what has been called the 'theory–practice' gap. It is all too easy to separate out the 'knowledge' elements of nursing from the 'skills and attitudes' element. What happens, then, is that nurses learn a lot about the *theory* of nursing and about the *practice* of nursing but they do not seem to tie the two together. Throughout your training (and beyond it) it is essential constantly to relate theory to practice and vice versa. Planning your learning can help you do this.

These, then, are issues concerning *what has to be learned*. In this section, we have referred to the 'formal' element of learning: what you are required to learn in order to become a nurse. Alongside this formal aspect is what is sometimes called the 'hidden curriculum'. Apart from the syllabus of training, there is a whole range of things that you learn simply by working with other people in a hospital, clinic or community setting. The hidden curriculum is not part of your formal training. It includes those things that you learn in order to survive. Examples of some of the things that you may learn under this heading include:

- How colleagues prefer to be addressed.
- What various senior staff prefer you to do when working in their wards.
- What you should and should not do to keep people happy.
- What the hospital expects of you.
- What your teachers like you to say to them.
- How to pass your assessments first time.

The hidden curriculum is often more influential than the more formal one. We all have to 'learn the ropes' and to learn how to cope with 'how things *really* are' as opposed to 'how they *should* be'. Being able to distinguish between the formal and the hidden curriculum may be one route to marrying theory to practice. For the person who learns both can also learn to choose his or her own path through nursing by combining both informal and formal aspects of the discipline.

Then, there is the issue of *how* nursing is learned. It is important, at an early stage of training as a nurse, to become familiar with the teaching and learning strategies used in the college and in the clinical settings. We all learn in different ways. Some will learn best through formal lectures, others through 'doing' and others by reading about a topic. Nursing involves a lot of 'doing' and is often thought of as a 'practical' discipline. It is important to recognize, though, that it is also developing a large and diverse body of theoretical knowledge which can be conveyed through a number of teaching and learning methods. Some of these are discussed in the paragraphs below.

Finally, in this section, it is important to know what *assessment methods* will be used in the course that you are undertaking. Typically, assessment will be a mixture of your having to demonstrate practical ability and ability to work with ideas and theories. You are likely to undergo most of the following forms of educational assessment:

- Written tests and examinations
- The submission of essays and projects

- The completion of case studies
- Clinically based assessments of nursing, interpersonal and management skills

Become familiar, at an early stage, with each of these forms of assessment. Find out what *sorts* of tests and examinations you will have. Find out, too, what types of essays you are going to have to write. Check on the format for the clinical assessments. It is always better to know, in advance, the *structure* of these assessments methods. If you are clear about *how* you are going to be assessed, then *what* you are assessed *on* remains the only other thing on which you have to work.

How am I taught?

As we have suggested, most colleges of nursing use a variety of teaching and learning methods. In the following paragraphs we explore some of those that are more frequently used. Before you read on, stop and reflect for a moment on the teaching and learning methods that you have been used to up to now. Reflect, particularly, on the following questions:

- What type of teaching and learning experience did you *most like* at school?
- What type of teaching and learning experience did you *least like* at school?
- What was the most commonly used type of teaching method at your school?
- If you were asked how you learn best, what would you say?

Lectures

Nursing diploma courses often involve fairly large numbers of students. A familiar method of passing on information to larger groups of students is the lecture method. Most people are familiar with lectures and they usually involve a teacher or lecturer standing in front of the group and speaking to that group for a period of about 50–60 minutes. Good lecturers will use a range of methods of varying the way in which information is passed on and will use things like:

- A white or blackboard
- An overhead projector
- A flip chart
- Pictures
- Slides

The point of using such methods is not simply to brighten up the lecture. They are also used because different people learn in different ways. Some of us learn by listening to other people, but some learn through seeing visual images. This is what makes reading such an important medium.

Lectures are probably the most traditional means of teaching and they have a number of advantages and disadvantages. Here are some:

Advantages

- Large amounts of information can be given to large numbers of people.
- Good lectures can enable the lecturer to develop a theme or a series of ideas without interruption.
- Students do not have to feel that they are 'put on the spot'. They simply have to listen and take notes.
- Good lectures can help to clarify what is written in books and what is experienced in clinical settings.

Disadvantages

- Poor lectures can be boring.
- In general, lectures do not allow people to *interact*. Interaction is seen by modern educationalists as a fairly central element in the learning process.
- Lectures do not account for different people's levels of knowledge. Some people may be 'lost' in a lecture while others are hearing what they know already.

Some students really enjoy lectures while others hate them. However, they are a fact of most educational programmes and it is important to make full use of them. Here are some pointers towards using lectures to enhance your own learning:

- Decide whether or not you need to take notes. Do not assume that you *have* to take notes. Some people learn best simply by listening.
- If you *do* take notes, plan your note taking carefully. This issue is discussed in a later chapter. Whatever form of note taking you choose, do not try to take down everything that the lecturer says.
- Allow yourself to have 'time out' in a lecture. No one can concentrate for the full span of a lecture. If you can allow yourself a couple of minutes 'break' when more familiar material is being covered, you can come back to the lecture refreshed.
- If there is a period for asking questions at the end of the lecture, or during it, make full use of it. Do not feel that you are being judged by other students or by the lecturer. Instead, use the time to clarify and to make sure that you understand what is being said. Do not be embarrassed to ask questions.

Seminars

The seminar is also a popular teaching strategy. Here, students are invited to lead discussions with their peers. Usually, a programme of seminars is drawn up at the beginning of a term and each student gives one seminar during the course of that term. Sometimes, students give seminars in twos or threes and this can be less anxiety provoking. Many students find the *idea* of giving a seminar nerve racking (and the first one often *is*). Planning can help to make it less and so and there seems little doubt that well run seminars can be a useful way of sharing knowledge and of learning new information.

The traditional method of giving a seminar is for the student to read a prepared paper to his or her colleagues. After the paper, a discussion is held between the student, his or her lecturer, and the rest of the group. Increasingly, however, more informal methods of organization are being used. One of the most effective ways of running a seminar is as follows:

- The student prepares a handout or an overhead acetate with about six leading questions on the topic in hand.

- Each question is then discussed with the group of students and the discussion is led by the student giving the seminar.
- Key issues that arise out of the discussion are marked up on a black or white board or on a flipchart pad.
- At the end of the seminar, the student-leader summarizes the discussion and offers other group members a reading list based on the original topic.

The value of this approach is that it takes the pressure off the individual student and it encourages all members of the group to take part. Many educationalists feel that adults learn best when they are actively *involved* in their learning. Learning, for them, is not a passive activity but one which involves the whole person. The seminar which is almost completely interactive is likely to be both more useful and more popular with other students. Like lectures, there are advantages and disadvantages:

Advantages

- Everyone, in turn, takes part in the teaching and learning process.
- You have to learn to organize your material so that others understand it.
- You can easily get feedback from others about your own knowledge base.

Disadvantages

- Not everyone likes getting up in front of their group and talking.
- The format allows people to wander off the topic unless the seminar is tightly structured.
- Some people get bored by other people's presentations.

Tutorials

Tutorials are a form of one-to-one learning. In the traditional tutorial, the student meets with his or her tutor to discuss a particular topic. Often, such tutorials may focus on a recently marked essay. The aim of the tutorial is to offer a more intensive opportunity to learn through discussion. Some tutors prefer to hold small *group* tutorials in which three or four students meet with him or her to discuss a particular topic. Key points in making good use of tutorials are these:

- Go prepared. Read the recommended reading before a tutorial and do not try to 'play it by ear'.
- Challenge your tutor. Do not take everything that he or she says as being the last word on the topic. Be prepared to disagree with him or her and to argue your case.
- Enjoy your tutorial and try to relax. In a one-to-one tutorial, you are not in competition with other people and you are not being compared with them. Take advantage of being able to quiz your tutor.

Advantages

- One-to-one learning with a tutor.
- You have the chance to discuss things in private as opposed to in front of your friends and colleagues.

Disadvantages

- You can be put on the spot if you have not prepared your work.
- You might not like the person with whom you have the tutorial.

Experiential learning

We are learning, all of the time. Experiential learning can refer to at least two things:

- Learning from living and working
- Learning through interactive teaching methods

Learning from living and working

Nursing, as we have noted, is a practical and interactive process. The fact that we deal, daily, with lots of different sorts of people is educational in itself. Other people are teaching us both formally and informally. The point is to *notice* that this is going on. It is quite easy to go through life without noticing what we are learning. The trick, if there is one, is to 'stay awake', to notice what is going on in the present moment and to reflect on what has happened, afterwards. Here is a simple example. Put down this book for a moment and reflect on your thoughts and feelings about it so far. Now think about how it compares to other books you have read. Now think, in a more general sort of way *what* books you have read. As you allow your focus of attention to expand in this way, you can begin to make links between what you are doing in the present and what has happened in the past. The point is that this will *not* happen unless you *choose* it to happen. The way to learn from living and working is to continue to notice what happens to you and to continue to reflect on what happens.

Learning through interactive teaching methods

In recent years, there has been a considerable shift towards lecturers and teachers using interactive teaching and learning methods. Here are some of the methods that you may come across in your college of nursing:

- Role play
- Pairs activities
- Small group discussions
- Psychodrama
- Stress reduction techniques

All of these sorts of methods involve a high degree of participation on the part of students. Not everyone likes this and some people find teaching methods such as role play take a bit of getting used to. However, the evidence seems to suggest that most people do learn if they are involved in what is happening in any given teaching session. Here are some suggestions about how to make best use of the experiential learning methods that may be used in your college:

- Take part as much as possible. If you feel embarrassed at first, allow yourself to feel this way but carry on anyway. As you get more used to expressing your point of view, the process will become more comfortable.
- Take some risks. If you are usually shy and reserved, pretend, for a little while, that you are not! If volunteers are called for, put yourself forward.
- Keep your attention focused on what is happening in the group. Notice other people's reactions to group activities.

- Learn to listen to other people. You can learn a lot from what other people have to say. Do not feel that you necessarily have to agree or disagree with what they have to say. Just accept, sometimes, that this is *this* person's point of view.
- Do not try to take notes during an interactive session. If you want, jot down some thoughts and feelings *after* the session. If you want to, structure these notes under headings. The following headings can be helpful, here:

  - type of activity
  - aim of the activity
  - immediate reactions
  - links with nursing practice
  - links with theory
  - reading to be done·

Advantages

- You *have* to take part and therefore you learn through doing.
- You are encouraged to reflect on your own, as well as on others', experience.
- Experiential learning methods can be more interesting than more formal ones.

Disadvantages

- Not everyone likes taking part in learning in this way.
- You may have to share some of your own ideas and this may make you feel a bit uncomfortable.

Planning your time

Planning is essential if you are going to keep up. As we have noted, on a nursing course, you have to divide your time in at least three ways between practical work in the clinical setting, educational activities in the college of nursing and your own social life and free time. Unlike many students, you do not simply have to learn from books and write essays, you also have to do an almost full-time job as well. First, you need to keep a diary. Buy one before the beginning of the year and fill in all the dates that you *know* before the year starts. For example, you may be able to fill in the following:

- The dates of blocks of study in the college
- Your ward or other clinical placements
- Your holidays

Once you have done this, you are able to see, immediately, which are likely to be the busiest parts of the year. Also, if you can, make a note of the assignments (essays or projects) that you are going to have to do. Again, this will give you a clear idea of what your academic workload is going to be like. The process of structuring your time in this way is also likely to give you a sense of being able to cope better. Whenever things get difficult, *structure* helps.

Once you have got into the habit of keeping a diary, use it all the time. Carry it with you and do not be tempted to keep two diaries – one in your room and one that you carry with you. If you do this, something is bound to get left out of one or the other. Instead, buy a diary that is big enough for you to make notes in and to include sufficient details to allow you to know exactly what is happening at various points in the year.

Keeping to schedule

Next, you need to get into a habit of planning what you do on a day-to-day basis. A good strategy, here, is to make 'to do' lists. With these, you simply list, each day or each week, the things that have to be done in that time span. Get used to making these quickly and only ever work with *one*. Like the two diary situation, it is easy to have one to-do list in your pocket and another in your room. You can be sure that something important will be missing off the one you are using.

Also, get used to listing the things that you need to do under the following headings:

- What *must* be done.
- What *should* be done.
- What *could* be done if there is time.

You will see examples of this approach throughout the chapters in this book. These three headings can help you to rank your tasks. For example, if you are writing an essay, your list of 'musts', 'coulds' and 'shoulds' may look something like this:

Musts
Go to the library
Find references for essay
Brainstorm and outline essay (see Chapter 4 for details)
Write it
Hand in no later than Friday 16th January

Shoulds
Discuss ideas with Andrew and Sarah
Book computer for wordprocessing (see Chapter 7 for details)

Coulds
Ring up David and ask his advice
Go to other library at St Mary's

The 'must–should–could' approach works with both formal work for your course and with other life situations. You might use it, for example, to make decisions about arranging your finances or for organizing your social life. The more structure you can use, ironically, the more freedom that you have. The structure frees you to concentrate on the things that you have and want to do.

If you fall behind

Nobody's perfect and almost everybody gets behind at some point. The first thing to do is to *tell someone*. The real danger is that you struggle along trying to catch up with your work and getting more and more anxious. This, in turn, slows you down even more. First of all, go and see your tutor and explain the situation to him or her. Assert yourself a bit here and do not be nervous of asking for an extension for an essay submission or for a rearrangement of a seminar. Use this sort of assertion sparingly, though. Most tutors will give you one extension but not many will thank you for asking for two or three. Learn from your time-management problem and go back to your diary to see how you can avoid the problem in the future. If you *do* ask for an extension or a change of arrangements, make sure that your request is a reasonable one. One of us recently had the following conversation with a student which illustrates the problem of not asking for enough time:

Student: I need more time for your essay and I'm worried that I won't get it in on time.
Lecturer: How long do you need?
Student: Could I have until Thursday?
Lecturer: How much work have you already done on the essay?
Student: Well . . . not very much really.
Lecturer: Have you done an outline?
Student: No, not yet.
Lecturer: Do you think that you can really get it done by Thursday?
Student: No, not really.
Lecturer: Have another week. Hand it in on Thursday week – that should give you time to do the necessary research and to write it.
Student: OK. Thank you very much.

The problem and the solution are obvious. If you ask for time, make sure that you ask for enough. On the other hand, make sure that you do not ask for time, over and over again. Once you have agreed a re-scheduling, make sure that you stick to the new dates.

Planning checklist

The following are questions to reflect on when you consider planning your learning:

- How do I learn best?
- Have I made good use of the resources available to me?
- Am I clear on the differences between tutorials and seminars?
- Will I stick to my plans?
- Will I be able to have a social life alongside my studies?

Managing other aspects of your life

Student life is not all about studying. Other sections of this book discuss how to manage relationships, sexuality, being assertive and what to do when things go wrong. An essential and fairly urgent issue for most students, however, is how to manage *money*. Most students have to rely on grants and grants are never very large. On the other hand, some may be fortunate enough to obtain bursaries and these may be more generous. Either way, being able to organize the way you spend and save money is essential to survival. Many banks now have special student accounts which offer special overdraft facilities, cheque card and cheque book conditions. It is worth investigating different banks and building societies to see which can offer you the best facilities for managing your grant and any other income. Barclays Bank offer the following guidelines for students:

- Always plan your budget as carefully and as accurately as possible.
- Always ask for advice when you need it.
- Never sign any financial document without checking it thoroughly and taking independent advice if you are not sure.
- If you borrow, do not borrow from too many places at the same time. It is important that credit cards should be used responsibly and beware of store cards which can be an expensive form of credit.
- Always use the APR (annual percentage rate) to check which interest rate gives you the best deal. Always let you bank know if you get in to difficulties – they are there to help (Barclays Bank, 1992).

Summary of chapter

This chapter has described various strategies for learning that are commonly used in colleges of nursing. Not everyone will benefit from all of them. What is important is that you determine, quickly, how *you* learn and then to exploit the means by which you do. Also, you need to be *structured* in your approach to working and learning. Before you move on to the next chapter, take some time to think about the planning that *you* need to do, both in terms of your learning and work and in terms of your social life.

3

Finding information

Finding information
These are the things that you must *do:*
<ul><li>Become familiar with all of the learning resources that are available in your organization</li><li>Search for information in a systematic way</li><li>Keep a record of *how* you go about searching for information</li></ul>
These are the things that you should *do:*
<ul><li>Keep detailed records of what you read</li><li>Take notes during lectures and seminars</li><li>Read through the notes that you take and expand on them</li></ul>
These are the things that you could *do:*
<ul><li>Learn how to do computer literature searches</li><li>Use a computer to store information</li><li>Discuss the information that you find with colleagues and lecturers</li></ul>

Aims of the chapter

- To explore all aspects of information retrieval.
- To enable you to think about how you keep notes.

The abilities to find, store and retrieve information are central to the business of being a student. The principle could be taken further. Someone once defined an intelligent person not as one whose head was filled with knowledge, but someone who knew where to find information if he or she needed. Being able to bring together different sorts of information, quickly, will make an important difference to your work as a nursing student – particularly on the academic side of things.

Tutorial staff

The tutorial staff are there to guide you towards the information that is needed to help you to become a nurse. This may not always be apparent: some tutors are better in this respect than others. Seeing tutors as 'information sources' is a good way of looking at them. They are not necessarily there to teach you all there is to know about a particular topic. Indeed, they could not do this. They should, though, make it clearer where you can find the information. They can also help you to make sense of the information that you collect. It would be reasonable, then, to ask the following things of a tutor:

- That they explain principles to you
- That they supply up-to-date reading lists of books and papers that are readily available
- That they are prepared to answer your questions
- That they will, if necessary, help you to find the books and papers in question
- That they will be prepared to talk through the things that you read

Make full use of your tutors. Like everyone, they are usually busy, so respect the fact that they may not be able to see you *now*. Instead, get used to an appointment system and turn up, on time, to see them. Also, do not expect too much of them. They cannot possibly know every reference and every theory that exists on a particular topic.

Using the library

The library will usually be your first port of call in the search for particular books and articles. Here are some of the ways in which the library can help you. Not all libraries will have all of these facilities.

- Access to books, reports, articles, theses and dissertations
- A CD-ROM machine which will enable you to do computerized literature searches
- Bibliographies which will help you to locate particular publications and papers
- Staff who can guide you towards the information that you need
- A computer literature-searching facility. This feature may cost you money to use
- Photocopier
- Journal clubs
- Invited and guest lecturers

Most colleges and university departments offer induction courses in how to use the library. Do not take the attitude that 'once you've seen one library, you've seen them all'. Getting to know *this* library is essential. Different libraries are laid out in different ways. Also, libraries use various systems for classifying books. Make sure that you know the one that your library uses. Make sure, too, that you know the location of the following:

- The shelves containing books that you are likely to need
- The shelves containing journals, reports and bibliographies
- Theses and dissertations and back numbers of journals (often referred to as 'the stacks')
- Indexes, computer guides, the CD-ROM machine and other peripherals
- Study carrels or desks
- Photocopying machines and any required tickets for the use of these.

Make sure, too, that you are clear about how to get books out of the library, how many you can take out and for how long. Get to know the librarians and how exactly they can help you. Also, make sure that you get your books back to the library on time. Fines can soon add up and the longer you keep them over the 'due back by' date, the larger the fines. There are two other points to make here: do not be tempted to steal books and do not 'hide' books in other parts of the library for your own use.

Other resources

Information does not just come out of tutors, books and journals. There are numerous other ways to collect data which you can use in your college work and in your examinations. As we shall see, too, chance can play a part. Here are some other sources of information about nursing and the theory and research that surrounds it:

- Nursing colleagues on the wards and in the community
- Government reports
- Leaflets and booklets in GP surgeries and in clinics
- Computerized information in the form of databases and CD-ROM
- Television and radio programmes

Serendipity

Serendipity is the art of making pleasant and unexpected discoveries. Do not expect that all of your information will come from the expected sources. Stay open to other possibilities. When you are in the library, for example, browse through shelves other than the ones you normally browse. One of the authors of this book found a 'missing link' in his PhD research while looking at books in the linguistics section of a local public library. The fact is that by looking at the shelves in the library that you do not usually visit, you can make some startling and unexpected discoveries.

Read newspaper and magazines about topics other than nursing. Again, newspapers – and particularly newspapers published at the weekend – often contain articles that will address topics that you are studying in the college, yet the slant taken by a newspaper reporter or writer will often be different to the one you are used to.

Also, read novels. They can often give you insights into the human condition that textbooks and journal articles cannot. In the end, read everything you can. Some of the most important discoveries in science and in history have come about not through the logical working through of a discipline but by chance – often through a 'penny dropping' or 'ah-ha!' experience. Expect the unexpected and you can do much to encourage serendipity. It may be chance, but you can raise the likelihood of chance occurring!

Taking and keeping notes

Information does not stay in your head for very long. It needs to be recorded. Taking and keeping notes is an important part of collating information. There are at least two ways in which you can record notes:

- By using pads of paper and files
- By storing the information on a personal computer

Many people still feel that 'being a student' involves keeping masses of files that are full of paper. You can do it that way but bear in mind that, if you buy a computer, you can keep your notes on discs and have instant access to a wide range of notes. There is more information about buying and using a computer in Chapter 7.

Using paper and files

Most people like buying stationery. There is no research to prove this but you only have to look in any stationery chain-store at the end of August to see hoards of people choosing the right pad and the right file. Two principles apply in the buying of stationery for note-taking. First, think big. You are going to collect a lot of notes over a period of three or four years. Try to think what a collection of notes is going to look like at the end of the first year and buy files to suit that view. Many people start off by buying a thin A4 pad of paper and a single ring binder. Consider, instead, buying a pack of 'Jumbo' A4 pads and a pack of three or four lever-arch files. Also, buy a series of index cards that will allow you to divide up your notes.

Consider, also, whether or not you will take rough notes and write-up the notes that you take during lectures. There are at least two views on this. Some people feel that it is a waste of time to write notes twice. Those people are of the view that you should aim at taking notes that can go straight into your files. If you choose this approach, make sure that you can develop a note-taking system that is clear and that you can read your notes once you have taken them.

Other people are of the view that it is useful to write-up rough notes as a memory-jogging aid. Those people feel that the process of copying out notes into more elaborate and detailed paragraphs helps in the learning process. Do not, however, simply rewrite what you have taken down in the lecture. That is a waste of time. If you decide to take 'rough notes' during a lecture and then rewrite them for you file, *add* to the lecture notes. Make sure that the notes you include as your 'final draft' are augmented by the things you have read about the topic in question. Add references to books and articles and to research papers. In this way, your final notes can serve as a useful guide to revision.

Whatever you decide, make sure that the notes that you take are *useful*. Do not simply take notes because you feel that you *ought* to. Many students have files bursting with notes and handouts which never get looked at again. This means that you need to be *selective* about your note-taking. You may, for instance, take notes for *some* lectures and just listen to others, without jotting anything down. Many students feel that they are *obliged* to take notes and the first experience of sitting through a lecture without writing anything down can be unnerving. However, there is a view that we cannot do two things at once: we cannot, easily, listen to a person talking and take down what he or she is saying, as well. If you are confident about the *background* to a lecture, consider just listening. Also, you may want to try jotting down notes *after* the lecture, rather than during it. The main point, here, is that there are no once-and-for-all principles when it comes to note taking. Some students find it useful, others do not; some like to take notes at every lecture, some prefer to be selective; some try to write down most of the lecture (perhaps using a form of shorthand), others are content to jot down key words or phrases. Find out how you work best. Discuss with your friends how *they* keep notes and then study your own learning style.

There are numerous ways of getting the notes down on paper in a form that you will be able to read later. Here are just two methods: the 'spider web' and the 'alternating paragraphs'.

The spider web style of note taking invites you to think laterally. You start with the title of the lecture in the *centre* of your note pad and you add 'spines' to the central idea, as the lecturer develops his or her points. You then add further 'spines' to each of the initial ones. In this way, you develop a complex 'web' of ideas that covers the page. Figure 3.1 offers an example of the spider web formation.

A second approach to note taking involves laying out your notes in such a way as to allow each topic a new and clearly marked paragraph. Figure 3.2 illustrates this form of note taking. You start the first paragraph of your notes at the left hand margin and alternating ones at the middle of the page. If you use this approach you can work quickly through your notes, when you revise, and find the section that you want.

Storing information on a personal computer

More and more people are using personal computers to help them with their work. If you have one or are considering buying one, there

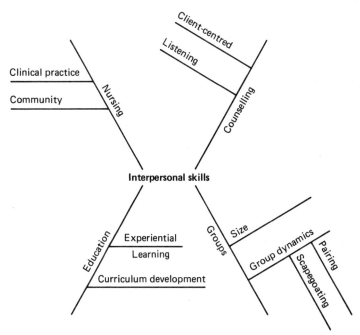

Figure 3.1 Spider web style of note taking

is no reason why you should not use it to help you keep notes. In Chapter 7, we discuss the questions of what sort of computer to buy and how to use one efficiently. Here, we just make some suggestions about how to organize note keeping on a computer.

First, make sure that you are thoroughly familiar with the idea of using directories and sub-directories. These are rather like the sub-dividers in a filing cabinet and they help you to organize your notes. Open a new directory for each topic that you study. Bear in mind that you can only use up to eight letters to name a directory. Thus you may have directories that read as follows:

- Biology
- IPS (interpersonal skills)
- Nursing
- Practs (practical nursing skills)
- Refs (bibliographic references)
  and so on.

Then, within each of these directories, consider keeping files that are recognizable by date. Thus, your files in the 'Nursing' directory may look like this. (Remember that you can only use eight letters or numbers to name a directory and an extension of a further three letters or numbers.)

- 120392 (12th March 1992)
- 040492 (4th April 1992)
  and so on.

Alternatively, you may prefer to give your notes descriptive names. You can use the three letter extension to highlight particular *types* of notes. Here is an example:

- Roy1.lec (Lecture notes on Roy's Model of Nursing, part one. The 'lec' extension indicates that the file contains lecture notes.)
- Rogers2.lec (Lecture notes on Rogers' Model of Nursing, part two)
- Rogers.ess (Notes for an essay on Rogers' work. The 'ess' extension indicates that the file contains an essay or notes for an essay)
  and so on.

The main point about organizing a set of computer notes is to be systematic. You do not want to have to spend hours searching for lost files that you know are on the computer somewhere. Organize your hard disc into directories (and sub-directories if necessary) and then be consistent about the way that you name files.

Perhaps the most important thing to remember about computer notes is that you *must* back them up to a floppy disc. Hard discs fail. When they do, there is every chance that your work will be lost. If you know where to go and you have the money, certain computer firms can sometimes recover data from damaged hard discs. The process is not recommended. Instead, make sure that you have a copy, on floppy discs, of everything that is on your hard disc. The test question is this: if your hard disc failed this afternoon, would you lose anything that you could not replace? If the answer is 'Yes', then you need to do some more backing up. Various programs are available that allow you to do incremental backups. This is to say, they will recognize which files have already been backed up and which ones are new. They then backup your new work to floppies. You can use one of these programs at the end of any given working session on the computer. Do not be lulled into a false sense of security. Do not work late into the night and then be tempted to leave the backing up to the next day. The chances are that you will not get round to it. Also, it is easy to slip into the habit of taking a chance and leaving backing up altogether. One of us did this until he lost the whole of two chapters of a book by pressing the wrong buttons. The chapters were gone forever and there was nothing for it but to sit down and rewrite them. After that, he did regular backups.

Information checklist

The following are questions to reflect on when you consider finding information:

- Am I clear about what I *need* to know?
- Do I know where to find the information I need?
- Am I systematic in my searching?
- Do I keep detailed notes and read these afterwards?
- Am I happy to seek clarification from a lecturer or clinical colleague?

Summary of chapter

This chapter has explored the process of finding and recording information. This process is at the heart of student life. The more systematically you can explore any given domain, the more you will know about it and understand it. Start as you mean to go on: find out *where* to obtain information and record the information that you collect.

Interpersonal skills
Question: what are interpersonal skills? Wide range of skills involving people interacting with one another. Interpersonal skills covers both one-to-one relationships *and* group relationships. Vital in nursing. All nursing interventions also involve interpersonal interventions.

Types of interpersonal skills
A number of types of interpersonal skills were discussed. Included in the discussion were:

- Listening
- Asking questions
- Responding
- Paraphrasing
- Reflecting

The importance of *listening* as the basis for all other interpersonal skills was emphasized. Listening to patients and relatives vital – and absence of *judgement* or *moralization* noted.

Interpersonal skills in nursing
See: Kagan, C. (1985) Interpersonal skills in nursing: research and applications, Kogan Page, London. Read first two chapters for next time. Prepare short seminar.

Figure 3.2   Using paragraphs for note taking

4

Keeping references

Keeping references
These are the things that you must *do:*   • Get into the habit of keeping references meticulously   • Be consistent   • Keep up to date by monitoring the latest journals
These are the things that you should *do:*   • Adopt one system for keeping your references and stick to it   • Review your method of keeping references from time to time   • Use your references for revising for end of year examinations
These are the things that you could *do:*   • Use a computer based system for keeping references   • Use the extensive range of library facilities available to you   • Keep a separate notebook in which you record where and when you have searched particular sections/subject areas of the library

Aims of the chapter

• To prepare you for taking references and using them successfully.
• To help you to identify different sorts of references and their relative merits.

- To assist to you to develop good study habits.

As a student you will have to gather a great deal of information in order to complete your written assignments and progress successfully through your course. In the last chapter we looked at some of the major sources of information that are available to you. Once you have found relevant information for completing a project you must use it effectively. One of the most effective ways of doing this is to develop a system for logging your reference material as you find it. At first, this may seem like a lot of unnecessary work. It is not. If you apply yourself and develop a systematic method for keeping references you will benefit greatly after a few short months on the course.

Why use references?

There are several reasons why you need to keep references during your time as a student. References will help you in the following ways.

To provide support for arguments

When you are writing an essay, preparing a seminar paper, or completing a much lengthier research dissertation, you will have to support your arguments with appropriate evidence. The type of evidence may vary. Sometimes you will use research papers, sometimes theoretical or discussion papers and perhaps on occasions you may use editorials to bolster your position. When you offer a view that is personal, then say so and try to provide a rationale for it.

To see how fields of information blend together

Another very important reason for using references is to enable new insights and understandings about a particular topic to be highlighted. Your perspective is a personal view of the world – so the references which you cull from the library when preparing your work will reflect your views. If you search for information in a diligent and imaginative way you may find new links between apparently diverse fields of study and express these in your work. This is why good literature review articles are so important and informative. Moreover, this is part of the 'cumulative' and discovery components of science.

To provide the reader with a chance to check your work

When you provide details about the literature you have used to build your arguments, you have in effect offered the reader a chance to check those references for themselves. You may have misrepresented a particular author, or referred to an author of which your tutor is unaware. By providing all the relevant details, you know that the reader can check your interpretations and representations for themselves, and this awareness will help to keep you on your toes and ensure that you are careful in the way in which you use references. It is all too easy, especially in an area which is new to you, to focus on a particular section of an article or book you have read, and miss critical points which your tutor will be very comfortable with. Be careful not to do this.

To communicate information with others

One of the main purposes for writing at all is to communicate with others. We use references in this communication process to keep others informed of current theoretical developments, debates and research findings. This is more true for lecturers and researchers, but the process is essentially the same. As a student you may find yourself in a position where you can communicate important information to professional colleagues, clients or fellow students. Until there is a major change in the organizational culture of institutions like hospitals, so that library study is an integral component of the professional nurses' work, students will be a very influential source of new ideas and developments. You will need to be competent in fulfilling this role of communication with others, even as a student.

To explore the known literature

As you complete course assignments and projects you will find you are being constantly bombarded with new ideas and long lists of references. You will have to find and read at least some of these if you are to understand each of the topic areas covered during your course. It pays to be organized and systematic. If you start keeping references early on in your course, you will not have re-search the same part of the library again and again as topics are revisited at a more advanced stage of your training. Keeping references will help you to cut down the amount of work you have to do later in the course.

Use of references

References can be used in different ways and for different purposes.

How many references are needed?

Students often ask, 'How many references do I need?' There is no simple answer to this. The more you read the greater the likelihood that you will be able to integrate this extensive reading into your work. However, some fields of study may not be well supported by publications. You may spend a great deal of time looking for relevant information and find that there is very little. In contrast, in other areas (for example the field of 'stress'), you may be overwhelmed by the vast range and depth of the literature which is readily available. What you will need, is a number of suitable references which support the general propositions in your work. These should reflect the main issues which you discuss.

   References should not be used as a type of 'cake decoration'. You should not write your project and then look around for things which seem to fit in nicely with your ideas. Nor should you squeeze in four or five references when one will suffice to make the point you wish to make. The 'quality' of the reference is important too (see section below).

Where do references go?

When you use a reference, place it at the end of a sentence to avoid breaking up the flow of your prose. If you put references in brackets in the middle of a sentence they will make the readability of what you have to say rather disjointed. Of course, sometimes you may have to mention an author in the middle or beginning of a sentence, but generally try to refrain from giving the name and date until the end of the sentence or section.

Which reference system is best?

There are two styles of referencing – The Harvard system and the Vancouver system – and these are described below. Both are correct but check which one your college prefers and use this preferred style in your work. If you are preparing your work for publication familiarize yourself with the reference style favoured by the journal you hope to get published in and make sure that your paper conforms to their wishes. If you do not they may return your work and refer you to their 'Guidelines for Authors'.

Quoting passages directly

Reference keeping can be especially useful when you encounter a powerful passage which you feel you could quote directly in your work. Be meticulous when noting down the particular passage and check it to ensure that you have copied it accurately. Note down all the relevant details about the book or articles – as you would for any reference – but also note the specific page number where the quotation may be found. Remember too that you may quote a maximum of 300 words only to keep in line with copyright laws.

Use only the 'best' passages. You may find that when you first begin to keep references systematically you may be tempted to note down lots of direct quotes. As you become more skilled in reading and analysing books and articles, you will become better at paraphrasing written material and find that you are much more selective in the things which you feel are 'quotable'.

Make sure that the passages you quote are 'linked' into the central issues you are discussing. You need to be clear therefore about what it is you want to say and avoid putting a 'string' of quotations together with no real structure to thread these into a clear and relevant argument.

It is okay to have your own opinions

It is perfectly acceptable to offer your own opinions or interpretations of material when writing your assignments. You cannot offer research for everything you may say. When you do this, however, try to ensure that you include some basis for these. It is very easy to slip into a style of writing which expresses your views on every second line of the text without offering an explanation as to *why* you think this or that is the case. Here is where you can begin to shore up your view by analysing, re-organizing or re-interpreting some of the reference material which you have used. Be wary, too, if you find yourself using lots of sentences which begin with phrases like 'I think', 'I feel', 'Everybody knows' and so on.

Types of publications containing references

When you search the library or have feedback from your tutor, you will quickly become aware of the fact that the papers and books which you use vary considerably. The quality and the nature of the audience for which these are published usually determines the type of paper or books which are produced. You need to be aware of the type of information you are gathering so that you can evaluate it fully and use it effectively. The following are some of the types of papers or articles you may find.

Research papers

These are the articles which report on the findings of original or replicated research. As a general rule, research papers are very informative and valuable as they provide you with the results of systematic investigations which report certain types of 'facts'. If the results of a number of research papers tell you that giving information to patients before surgery helps them to get better quickly, this is much more impressive than if someone merely expressed a 'belief' that this was so. Whatever the nature of the assignment you are working on, try to retrieve some research papers which will help to complete the project.

Theory papers

These papers do not report new research findings but may well use research to support particular theoretical frameworks which are offered in the paper. This is part of the cyclical process of research – theory–research–revise theory. The theories described are often 'hunches' about a given topic. These theories can then be tested out by gathering information (in a systematic manner) and this can lead to the acceptance, rejection or revision of the theory. Many papers which are in effect reviews of the literature on a specific topic, provide a new theoretical slant on a given topic. Because new insights or ideas are often generated in theory papers, new gaps in the literature will emerge and these have to be explored fully by researchers if these new ideas are to hold up over time.

Opinion papers

Another important source of information may be gleaned from opinion papers. A good example here is the 'editorial' which many journals and magazines include in their publications. These can be written without recourse to any further source – they are just the 'opinion' of the writer. You must be careful about using these as support for your opinion when you write your assignments. Just because a famous author states a personal view does not mean that this view is accurate. It is merely an opinion not a fact. The author may have a particularly strong view about the topic and he or she may have a particular axe to grind, so be careful when using this type of paper in your work.

Types of books

Books vary too. Here are some of the sorts of books which you will encounter when preparing your assignments.

Monographs

This is a paper or book which deals with a single subject area or part of a subject area. Many of these report research findings from particular subject areas and this type of reporting is usually done in great detail. Monographs enable you to become very familiar with the subject areas and to consider various aspects of that area – be they methodological, theoretical or practical issues – by referring to this single source. Research monographs are popular among researchers who find details about the research which may not have been published in the shorter research journal papers.

Edited volumes of research reports

These are texts which are edited for consistency, clarity and coherence. They are, in effect, extended research journal papers which contain many more details about the methodology and the implications of the research for practitioners, researchers and educators. Edited volumes of research may take one of two basic forms. One approach is to link the chapters by 'methodology' – in this case the volume is more concerned with the theoretical approach used to guide the research and/or specific research method used for the studies. The other approach is to link the chapters by 'content area' – here the specific subject area is explored by different researchers using a variety of theoretical perspectives, approaches to research and research tools.

Single topic textbooks

These textbooks contain information about a single subject area such as 'stress', 'pharmacology' or 'statistics'. However, they usually explore a whole range of issues related to the given topic. It is important to note that such books may or may not rely on research findings as they communicate information. Often they will mix the opinions of the author with research from other authors so be careful when you choose to use these texts as reference material to support your points.

Multiple-topic textbooks

These books tend to provide you with baseline information which you will need to get a handle of given subject areas. In a basic textbook of psychology for example you will find that it covers different topics such as: memory, social development, learning theory, consciousness, intelligence, motivation, social perception and social influence. Single topic textbooks are available on all of these topics so this general textbook will naturally be somewhat limited. Nevertheless, it may be suitable for your needs. Try to identify what has been put forward by the author as his or her ideas and whether or not these are backed up by appropriate research findings.

Examples of referencing styles

The examples of referenced passages, in this section, illustrate how the same piece of writing can be referenced using the Harvard method and the Vancouver method. Remember to check which style of referencing you are required to use and then learn to use that style properly. It is important not to mix the two styles.

Example of the Havard referencing system

Psychiatric nurses play an important psychotherapeutic role in the mental health care team. In the general field, nurses are often called upon to play out a counselling or supportive role (Tschudin, 1991). In recent years, there has been an accent on the development of interpersonal skills in nurse training and education, particularly in the UK (Kagan, 1985; Kagan, Evans and Kay, 1986). There has also been an emphasis in the literature on the use of experiential learning methods as the means of developing such skills (Dietrich, 1978). In this paper experiential learning is explored through the literature. Experiential learning and experiential learning methods have wide application in the fields of both psychiatric and general nursing.

References

Dietrich, G. C. (1978) Teaching of psychiatric nursing in the classroom. *Journal of Advanced Nursing*, 3, 525–534.
Kagan, C. M. (ed) (1985) *Interpersonal Skills in Nursing: Research and Applications*. Croom Helm, London.
Kagan, C. M., Evans, J. and Kay, B. (1986) *A Manual of Interpersonal Skills for Nurses: An Experiential Approach*. Harper and Row, London.
Tschudin, V. (1991) *Counselling Skills for Nurses*, 3rd Edition. Baillière Tindall, London.

Example of the Vancouver referencing system

Psychiatric nurses play an important psychotherapeutic role in the mental health care team. In the general field, nurses are often called upon to play out a counselling or supportive role. In recent years, there has been an accent on the development of interpersonal skills in nurse training and education, particularly in the UK.[1] There has also been an emphasis in the literature on the use of experiential learning methods as the means of developing such skills.[2,3,4] In this paper experiential learning is explored through the literature. Experiential learning and experiential learning methods have wide application in the fields of both psychiatric and general nursing.

References
1. Tschudin, V. (1991) *Counselling Skills for Nurses*, 3rd ed. Baillière Tindall, London.
2. Kagan, C. M. (ed) (1985) *Interpersonal Skills in Nursing: Research and Applications*. Croom Helm, London.
3. Kagan, C., Evans, J. and Kay, B. (1986) *A Manual of Interpersonal Skills for Nurses: An Experiential Approach*. Harper and Row, London.
4. Dietrich, G. C. (1978) Teaching of psychiatric nursing in the classroom. *Journal of Advanced Nursing*: 3, 525–534.

Keeping a reference database

We strongly recommend that you learn to use a computer effectively in your education on a daily basis. Both of us use computers everyday and have found them to be invaluable. However, you may not be convinced of the value of using a computer. Or you may not have the resources to purchase your own hardware at the moment. Moreover, suitable computer facilities in your particular institution may not be fully operational at the moment. You can still develop a system for keeping references without a computer but the computer has added advantages.

An index card reference system

This is the manual equivalent of the computer based system. You will need to purchase a box of index cards with alphabetic inserts which allow you to store your references alphabetically. Index cards come in different sizes but we think the larger format (20 cm by 12.5 cm) is best. You also need a box for keeping these safely and tidily. For each article or book that you read you *must* make out a new reference card if the material is at all relevant to your studies or assignments. Each card should have the following details:

For books
- Author
- Date
- Title
- Edition
- Publisher
- Place of publication

For articles
- Author
- Date
- Title
- Volume number
- Part number (if any)
- Page numbers

A summary of relevant points made in the publication and any passages which you wish to quote directly should also be listed on the

Abbott, P. and Wallace, C. (Editors) (1990) *The sociology of the caring professions*. Falmer Press, London.

This is a very interesting edited volume which looks at the following issues:
- The professions of social work and nursing
- Some of the historical developments of these groups
- The role of women in society and gender differences
- The push for professionalisation of these groups

On the issue of *caring as women's work* they state:

'... caring work is often seen as women's work and closely identified with what women are supposed to be doing for their families in any case' (p.5).

Figure 4.1   An example of a completed index card

card. Remember if you include direct quotations to include the page number where that passage may be found.

Place a 'key card' at the front of the box of cards which reminds you what each card refers to. This will enable you to track down important references by specific subject area. As you become more proficient in the use of the card system you will find that you note down which subject areas each particular reference is relevant to and cross reference these. Some of the references may be applied to different areas. The example in Figure 4.1 could refer to several different study 'areas'. The reference could be used when you are exploring the following sorts of issues: professional socialization, women and men in nursing, caring in nursing, sociology of nursing and the role of the caring professions. In this instance you need to identify the areas that the reference could apply to even though you may only wish to focus on one specific application for the moment. The other areas may be relevant for some later assignment or for your revision.

Because all of the references are stored alphabetically, you can easily find any card so long as you have the name of the author you are looking for. Figure 4.2 is an example of the type of key card which should be kept in the front of the index box:

Key card

Caring in nursing

Watson, 1979, 1985.
Briggs, 1972.
Griffin, 1980, 1983.
Morrison, 1992.

Psychological care of patients

Wallis, 1987.
Nichols, 1985.
Hyland and Donaldson, 1989.
Hall, 1990.
Morrison, 1992.

Qualitative interviews – purpose, design, analysis

Kvale, 1983.
Giorgi, 1975, 1985.
Adler and Adler, 1987.

Figure 4.2   An example of a key card layout for storing your references

Computerized reference databases

If you have a computer, you may want to keep your reference collection on it. You have two options here: you can either list all your references in a single, wordprocessor file, or you can store them in a database program.

The simplest approach is the first one. You simply open a wordprocessing file and then put your references into it, in the form of paragraphs, as you collect them. If your wordprocessor has a 'sorting' facility, it does not matter what 'order' you type them in. Once you have put in new references, you get the program to sort the entire list into alphabetical order. Here is an example of what your file will look like.

Brown, P. J. (1991) *Essential Biology*. Arnold and Smith, London.
Smith, D. (1992) *Nursing for Professionals*. Chapman and Hall, London.
Watson, P. (1990) A study of the way in which pressure sore care has been conducted in three London teaching hospitals. *Journal of Nursing Studies*: **2**, 34: 36–45.

There are many advantages to this approach to storing references. First, you can add new ones to the file very easily. Second, you can easily 'cut and paste' references from you list, straight into your essay or project. Third, the whole system is very easy to use and administer. If you feel that you will not be collecting huge numbers of references, this system may suit you.

The second approach is to use a ready-written database program. There are at least three sorts of these:

- A bibliographical database program
- A flat file database program
- A free-form database program

The bibliographical database program is one that is specially written for recording references. Thus, the program is set up for you to enter names, dates, titles and publishers of books and the details of journal papers. Such programs are usually fairly easy to run and you can transfer references from your wordprocessor into the program and export references into you essays and projects. The problem with using such a program is that it may not be possible to set it up *exactly* as you would like it.

This is where a flat file database program may be useful. This sort of program is flexible and works on the principle of 'forms and fields'. A 'form' is the equivalent of a single card, on which you keep the details of your reference. A 'field' is a space on that form in which you store specific details (author, date, title, publisher). Figure 4.3 is an example of a form, laid out with the appropriate fields.

Before you can use a database of this sort, you must first determine what fields you need and how *long* each of the fields will be. The best way to do this is to draw an example form, on paper, before you switch on the computer. You also need to make sure that each of your fields is long enough to contain the longest piece of text you are likely to put in it. Some flat form database systems insist that you can insert a maximum of 255 characters in any given field. This is usually long enough for most purposes but it does mean that you have to be careful about the length of the 'comments' that you write.

A flat file database system allows you to store you references systematically and allows you to design your own system to suit yourself. A number of commercial systems are available including *PC-File*, *Paradox* and *DataPerfect*. All take a little time to 'learn' and to get used to but such time is well invested.

The free-form database program overcomes the limitations of the flat file variety. The free-form program does not use forms and fields. Instead, you simply type all of your text into the program and then, at a later date, you search for the text you have typed. Thus, you may search for the word 'counselling' and the program will call up all the books and journal papers that have 'counselling' in the title. Alternat-

---

```
AUTHOR: {field 1}

DATE: {field 2}

TITLE: {field 3}

PUBLISHER: {field 4}

KEYWORDS: {field 5}

COMMENTS: {field 6}
```

Figure 4.3   Database form laid out with appropriate fields

ively, you may search for 'Smith, P. J.' and the program will show you all the entries you have made under that name. The free-form database does not offer such an 'organized' approach but it does mean that you can make entries such as shown in Figure 4.4.

Again, there is a variety of free-form database programs available, such as *Memory Mate* and *Info Select*. We have used Memory Mate to store a wide range of references on our own computers, both at work and at home. One of the bonuses of both Memory Mate and Info Select is that they are also 'Terminate and Stay Resident' programs. That is to say that they can be made to 'pop up' over any other program you are using. Thus, you may be working in your wordprocessor and you can call up Memory Mate to search for a particular reference. You can then 'cut and paste' that reference from Memory Mate directly into your wordprocessing file. You can then 'close down' Memory Mate and return to work on your original document. This sort of flexibility makes free form databases ideal for storing references that are varied in length.

Whatever database system you decide to use, one thing is vital: you *must* make backup copies of your data files. As you add references to your database, make sure that the file you enter the references in is backed up to floppy disc.

{Entry 1}
Smith, P. J. 1992 Counselling for Health Care Workers, Black and Little, London.
   This is a useful, introductory text on counselling. My copy of it is at home but there are other copies in the college library.

{Entry 2}
Davies, D. 1988 Primary Nursing and the Critical Care Nurse, Andrews, Edinburgh.
   Davies' book offers useful definitions of primary nursing. Use it for the 'nursing' essay in the second year. Consider buying this one. Note, particularly, the passage on page 62:
   'Although primary nursing is not a new concept, the idea and the practice has taken about 10 years to become established in the UK. There are still those who doubt that it can be used in the critical care field. '

Figure 4.4   Example of a free-form database entry

References checklist

The following are questions to reflect on when you consider working with references:

- Have I explored different ways of keeping and quoting references?
- Have I started a reference database?
- Is my reference database up to date?
- Have I used references effectively in my written work?
- When I have found out new information, have I conscientiously summarized it in the reference database?

Summary of chapter

This chapter has considered the question of how to record and store information about books and papers that you have referred to or read. It is vital that such a database of information is kept up to date and accurate. You may want to use cards or you may want to use a computer database: the point is to use a system that works for you.

5

Writing essays

Writing essays
These are the things that you must *do:*   • Visit the library to find material   • Make a plan   • Allow yourself sufficient time to complete the essay on time
These are the things that you should *do:*   • Read extensively around the topic   • Use a wordprocessor or typewriter   • Make several drafts
These are the things that you could *do:*   • Get the essay laser printed   • Discuss your views with fellow students and tutors   • Rewrite the essay in the light of constructive feedback from your tutor

Aims of the chapter

• To help you to make an effective plan for your essays.
• To outline the way in which you should structure your written work.

- To enable you to get good marks for your essays while in college.
- To equip you with some of the psychomotor skills needed to perform well under written examination conditions.

Writing essays is an important and valuable aspect of the educational process. It is also an integral part of a student's existence. When you come to college for the first time you may be surprised at the level of anxiety which students generate as they prepare to hand in their early attempts at essay writing. Moreover, students spend a great deal of time finding ways of putting off the business of getting down to writing up their essays. There is always something more interesting and more fun to do. However, even for the most relaxed of students, the inevitable happens and essays have to be produced if you are going to stay on the course of study upon which you embarked and achieve a professional qualification.

Essay writing can help you to: identify your own particular strengths and weaknesses and to take appropriate corrective action; organize your thinking and develop your own views and opinions about the topics under consideration; prepare to tackle unseen examination questions in which an essay format answer is required; revise for examinations.

Planning your essay

As soon as you get the title of your essay go to the library and start looking for material which may be relevant. This provisional scan will help you to draw up an effective essay plan which you can put to work. A good plan is absolutely essential if you want to get good marks for your essays. Remember too that essays can also form part of your end of year marks, so working hard on your essays can help to send you into end of year examinations with marks in the bank. A good essay plan has the following features (see Figure 5.1):

Introduction

An introduction sets the scene and maps out the basis for your discussion. It highlights the most significant points in a succinct fashion. The introduction should usually be written last. When you

Question: What interpersonal skills might students use in working with patients and how might they learn those skills?

Essay plan: word limit: 1500 words

Interpersonal skills
- A description of what the term 'interpersonal skills' means
- Outline of the essay
- Interpersonal skills in nursing: a short review of the research and literature
- Specific examples of interpersonal skills when working with patients:
  - Basic social skills: introductions, non-verbal communication etc.
  - Listening
  - Basic counselling skills
  - Assertiveness skills

Learning interpersonal skills
- Description of what 'learning' means
- Brief description of teaching and learning methods
- Nurses as adults: adult learning methods
- Learning interpersonal skills:
  - Experiential learning
  - Role play
  - Learning in the clinical setting
  - Learning from reflection
  - Learning from everyday life

Summary and conclusions
- Review points of essay and indicate what has been discussed.
- Raise issues for future:
- Nurses need further training in interpersonal skills
- Nurses need to monitor their own interpersonal skills.

Figure 5.1 Example of an essay plan

have covered all the relevant aspects of the essay you will be better able to highlight what is absolutely critical and mention these points in the introduction to grab the reader's attention early on.

Statement of content

You will need to be able to state clearly what the main points of the essay are in simple, straightforward sentences or phrases. You may find initially that you have lots of apparently relevant points to make so try to rank these in order of importance.

Development of the main content areas

When you look carefully at the provisional ideas you have generated you will see that they can be regrouped into different content areas. When you have done this you will find that you can begin to write short paragraphs about each of these. In this way you can develop the plan for your essay in this rough form.

Support for arguments

Be careful to ensure that you offer support for your arguments. As you map out the development of your main points avoid making rash and unsupported statements. Ask yourself if the things that you say can be supported by suitable research literature or logical and coherent reasoning.

Summary and conclusion

Your plan should have a conclusion which highlights the main issues in the light of the detailed discussion which you have offered.

Essential features of a good essay

Answers the question

A good essay answers the question that is asked. You must stick to the point and avoid going off at a tangent.

Clarity of style

If you are sure about what it is you want to say then clarity will not be a problem. Confused and woolly thinking leads to an unclear style of writing and confused prose. Use everyday language. Use short sentences and short paragraphs and avoid jargon and slang. If you can say something in one sentence rather than a page then say it in one sentence.

Logical structure

A logical structure is essential if you want to write clearly and effectively. Imagine that your tutor knows very little about the subject area and write in way which will allow him or her to follow the flow of the arguments as a novice. A good test here is to ask a friend, colleague or spouse to read your essay and see if they have followed the structure which you have adopted. If they have not, then you may need to restructure the skeleton framework within the essay. This is a good test too for all the other facets of writing.

Appropriate use of references

Use references appropriately. Do not wait till you have finished the essay and then look for references to 'fit in' to make the essay look right. Do not add references just to increase the size of the reference list. These tactics are often pretty transparent. Only use references where they add support for your arguments or where they provide the essential details which are needed to make a particular point.

Critical awareness and not just description

A good essay, even one in which description is a key feature, should show evidence of your critical awareness of the area being described. To do this you need to be able to stand back from the essay and points made in it and look objectively at what has been said by you and by the authors of the references you have included. A critical awareness of the topic shows the reader that you have begun to think about the area in a more informed and professional manner. This is discussed in more detail, below.

Complete reference list

If you have kept a record of the references you have used in your essay you will be able to produce a comprehensive list of references at the end of your essay. This is an essential feature of a good essay. The references should be listed either alphabetically or numerically, depending on which style of referencing you are using. Make sure that you do not omit any of these and that all relevant details are included. (See the section on referencing in previous chapter.)

Writing to deadline

Keep to the deadline which the tutor has set unless it is absolutely impossible. If you have planned and timetabled your work you should be able to meet the deadline. If you must ask for an extension then make sure you have a genuine reason for asking. One of the major problems of pushing back work is that the deadlines for other essays or projects get nearer, so you may be faced with even more work and a shorter time in which to do it. Make sure you keep up to date with your work schedule.

Correct number of words

Stick to the word limit which the lecturer has set for the essay. Do not under write or over write. If you find that you are worried about how to fill the pages then you probably have not done enough background reading or are not familiar enough with the material. Go back to the library and find more reading material. If, on the other hand you cannot seem to keep to the allocated word limit, then review your plan and trim it down to ensure that you do meet the necessary number of words.

Use your library

Do not think that because you have one basic textbook in psychology that will be enough reading material for writing an essay on any aspect of psychology. You must use all the resources at hand. Go to the library with the attitude of finding a wide range of material which you could use to answer the specific question which has been set in the essay. When you are in the library make sure that you are fully aware of the numerous ways in which you can find information (CD-ROM, computer catalogue, the librarian, the journal room and so on).

Tips on writing

Read the question carefully. Look for specific clues in the question which will indicate the sorts of things which the lecturer or examiner is looking for. Key words or phrases may include some of the following:

- Discuss . . .
- Write an account of . . .
- Explain . . .
- Compare and contrast . . .
- Critically evaluate . . .
- Evaluate . . .
- Describe . . .

These key words or phases should be kept in mind when you set about producing an outline plan for the essay. They tell you if the essay is to emphasize description, discussion or some form of evaluation. As you put together your plan keep referring back to the original question and the specific phrases that tell you what is required. If you are not sure whether your ideas at relevant, then bounce some of your ideas off a colleague, a friend or your personal tutor. It is easy to get side tracked so take care. Often new ideas which seem appropriate for the discussion are rather peripheral. A good essay shows that you have clearly understood the question.

Allow sufficient time

This is crucial. You will not be able to produce good essays if you leave all you preparation and library research up until the night before the essay deadline and then stay up until 2 a.m. writing the whole thing in one great burst. You may be faced with the prospect of having to prepare two or more essays by the end of the term so start working on them as soon as you can. Make out a mini timetable for going into the library and finding important references, identifying the most useful material, making notes and keeping records of what you read. Do not leave your writing till later. Get onto a wordprocessor and make early drafts of the essays as soon as you have drawn up a satisfactory plan. Remember that many other students will also be seeking out the material from the library and most people will leave it till late. Get in there early and get on with it.

Brainstorm

Brainstorming involves jotting down everything you can think of about a particular topic. Pay no attention to the relevance or otherwise of the things that you write down. The aim is to write quickly and without editing. The quicker you can work, the more ideas you generate. Here, for example, is a sample of brainstorming on the topic of *Health Care Assessment*:

- General Health Questionnaire
- General practitioners
- Self-care
- Physical and psychological care
- Spiritual care
- Health visitors
- Normal and abnormal behaviour
- Child care
- Who assesses
- Informal and professional assessment
- Home helps
- Research into health care
- Who assesses health care needs of the nation?
- Other countries
- Government policy
- Cultural considerations

Once you have generated a list of both relevant and less relevant items, work through the list, crossing out the irrelevances. Then, sort the items that you have left into a workable order. When you have done this, you are left with a ready-made structure for your essay. These basic ideas can then be developed in the body of your essay. The point of brainstorming is to allow your imagination the freedom to identify a wide range of ideas prior to writing out a more formal, essay structure. Also, the method encourages you to develop *original* ideas.

Once you get the hang of this technique you will probably find yourself using it all the time as a way of generating new ideas for your essays. This is particularly so in the early stages of planning your work.

Layout headings

When you have generated a large number of ideas through brainstorming, these will need to be organized or collated into some logical order or structure. This can be done by drawing up a series of heading or themes which, when laid out in a systematic fashion, will provide you with the basis of your essay. All you have to do then is to begin to expand the initial ideas which resulted from the brainstorming activity and form these into small sentences. This all sounds rather simple and mechanical but you will be surprised at the results when you have tried out these stages for yourself and produced a couple of essays for your lecturers. Make notes under headings.

Discuss with colleagues and lecturers

Sometimes even after reading widely around a particular topic you may find yourself at a loss as to where to start or what exactly is required. This may be especially true at the beginning of a new course when you are unsure about the particular parameters of the course or how a particular lecturer likes his or her essays written. Try to find out if there is a specific department format for essay writing or if individual lecturers recommend a certain style and conform to these. If you do get stuck, talk to your fellow students or your personal tutor. Bounce your initial ideas off these people and listen to their responses. Make notes after you do this so that you do not neglect any important points they may make. Carefully review your essay plan in the light of these discussions and do not be afraid to accept or indeed reject their advice.

Read extra material

Often, students as a group seem to hand in very similar essays. Do try to read widely and find relevant material which other students may not have uncovered in their search of the available literature. One of the characteristics of a good essay is the appropriate use of material which other students have not spotted in the library. To do this of course you will need to have allowed yourself enough time to visit the library and dig this out.

Getting down to it

Often the biggest problem students face when writing essays is the actual 'getting down to it'. You may have done all the reading and made a good plan but then you have to *write* something. Most people have experienced this problem – faced with a blank sheet of paper or a blank VDU with a flashing cursor. There is no escape you just have to get on with it. Write something – anything just to get yourself moving. Set yourself a small goal – write a sentence, a paragraph, write out the references you are sure you are going to use. The secret is to get moving in the right direction. This is where wordprocessing really comes into its own. Over a short period of time you can produce quite a polished essay in spite of the initial struggles. Make a first draft of the essay and be prepared to rework this into the polished article you hope it will be. There is no substitute for hard work.

Edit the drafts

Edit your early drafts for style, content, spelling, relevance to the specific question and so on and rewrite it or parts of it if necessary. This can be a painful process but if you want to get the best out of yourself you must be prepared to do this. If you have used a wordprocessor the task will be a lot less painful. When you are reasonably happy with the end product, print out a good copy and then leave it aside for a few days and concentrate on some other project. After a couple of days proofread this again and do any final editing that seems necessary. You will be surprised how a short break away from your essay can help you to re-evaluate it more objectively.

Be prepared to accept feedback

Essay writing is a learning process so you must be prepared to accept constructive criticism from your tutor. You may feel that you have worked particularly hard to produce a great piece of work but your tutor may have other ideas. Listen carefully to what the tutor has to say so that you can re-evaluate your own work more effectively in the future. Do remember also that tutors are human, too, and sometimes they get it wrong.

Keep a copy of your essay

Always keep a copy of your essay just in case it gets misplaced. You can also use your essays as part of your programme of revision for the end of year examinations.

Developing critical skills in writing

It is not sufficient merely to write nor just to report what other people have said about a particular topic. Increasingly, nurse teachers are requiring that essays be *critical* as well as descriptive. In degree and higher degree courses it is essential that you are able to illustrate some critical ability in your work.

What does it mean to be critical? Sometimes, the word is used only in its negative sense: 'to criticize'. In writing, though, it can also mean to be *positively* critical, to evaluate or judge quality. Some examples of descriptive and critical writing may help here. The first extract, below, illustrates writing that is descriptive. It describes what other (imaginary) people have written about a topic. In the second extract, the words in italics illustrate the writer offering some critical commentary.

Example 1
Brown (1991) in a paper about his research into stress in nursing illustrates how nurses often respond badly to feedback from ward staff. This idea of nurses being sensitive is further supported by White (1989) and Green (1990). On the other hand, Black (1992) suggests that nursing is no more stressful than many other caring professions and that there is little evidence that nurses are more sensitive to criticism than any other health care workers.

If nursing *is* stressful, then it is important that we build in support systems to help them to cope. Davies (1990) suggests that all nurses should have mentors. Mentors are people who can offer both clinical and personal support.

Example 2
Brown (1991) in a paper about his research into stress in nursing illustrates how nurses often respond badly to feedback from ward staff. *However, Brown used a very small sample in his study and he tended to generalize from his findings to a fairly large degree. His paper does not offer sufficient evidence to support the idea that most nurses respond badly to feedback.* This idea of nurses being sensitive, however, is further supported by White (1989) and Green (1990). *Both of these writers carried out large-scale reviews of the literature and offer evidence from both research and the literature. On balance, their conclusion that nursing is stressful and that nurses are sensitive to criticism seems to be supported.* On the other hand, Black (1992) suggests that nursing is no more stressful than many other caring professions and that there is little evidence that nurses are more sensitive to criticism than any other health care workers. *Black's study is particularly useful as he used a qualitative approach to comparing the thoughts and feelings of nurses working with children with social workers who also work with young people. Although generalization from qualitative studies should be avoided, the anecdotal evidence that Black offers is useful to anyone searching for specific examples of work-related stress. However, given the limitations of his research method, Black may not be able to generalize about whether or not nursing is more or less stressful than other sorts of health care.*

If nursing *is* stressful, then it is important that we build in support systems to help them to cope. Davies (1990) suggests that all nurses should have mentors. *She expresses this as an opinion and her claim is not supported by research or by evidence from the literature.* Mentors are people who can offer both clinical and personal support.

Learning to write from a critical perspective involves the constant asking of certain questions. Examples of these questions are:

- What evidence does this writer offer to support his or her claims?
- Is the researcher justified in making these claims for his or her research?
- Are there other points of view that are not being covered in the papers and research reports that you have read?

Learning to write critically is an important educational skill. It helps you to think clearly and rationally about the topic in hand and will be of use not only in essay and project writing for your course but also later in your career when you write business reports, articles or even books. Try to cultivate the ability to think and write critically as a way of life. As you read papers, reports and books, ask the above questions of the person whose work you are reading.

What *not* to do

- Do not wait until the last minute. We cannot emphasize this point too strongly. You must allow yourself time for the continuous process of reading, writing and reviewing your essays until you are happy with the final draft.
- Do not write to impress, write to express. Be clear about what you want to say and just state that. Offer support for your ideas and demonstrate a critical awareness of the material.
- Do not go over the word limit. Avoid 'fillers' like: 'At this moment in time', 'All things considered' and so on which add little and use up the limited space which you have to convince the assessor that you understand the critical issues which relate to a particular essay question.
- Do not go off the topic. Keep a check on yourself to make sure that what you write is relevant for the essay and the specific questions which you have been asked to address.
- Do not make unsubstantiated claims. Reread every sentence in your essay if you want to avoid falling into this trap.
- Do not misquote. If you use quotations, use them sparingly and make sure you quote the source accurately. Even small changes in a quotation can change the sense of it and its appropriateness for your essay.
- Do not plagiarize. Plagiarism means copying someone else's words and putting them forward as your own. This is illegal. Do not do it under any circumstances. It is fine to read other people's work and paraphrase it in your own words while acknowledging the source. Plagiarism is one of the cardinal sins of academic life and educational institutions could ask you to leave the course if you offend.

Presenting your work

You should always present your work in the best possible light and the best way to do that is to have the work typed or wordprocessed and printed out on a laser printer. Typed essays should be clearly laid out on the page and double spaced. Each page should be numbered and the essay should have your name and the tutor's name written on the title page. This is the best way to produce your work but sometimes

you may have to write out your essay by hand. If you have to do this
then always ensure that you write neatly and clearly. The best policy is
to learn how to use a wordprocessor and then use it. A well presented
essay should have the following features:

- A title page which includes the name of the student, course details,
  and the name of the lecturer for whom the essay was written.
- A typed, double spaced script which is page numbered.
- A script in which the grammar, sentence structure and spelling has
  been checked. Most good wordprocessing packages have a spell
  checking facility.
- A logical scheme of headings and subheadings. This depends
  greatly on the preferred style of the individual lecturers who set the
  essay titles. Find out what each likes and conform to that
  structure.

Marking schemes

Essays can be marked in different ways. Some tutors prefer to
'impression mark' – what the tutor is looking for in an answer is not
made explicit. Rather, they read through your essay and mark it
according to what they find in it. They may, as they go, offer you
comments on style, use of evidence, referencing, presentation and so
on. They may also offer you short comments at the end of your paper
such as 'fine', 'satisfactory' or 'rather disappointing', or (more use-
fully) a crisp critique of your paper and a series of written comments.

Other tutors, 'criterion mark'. Before they start marking your
paper, they are clear about what your answer should contain. They
will allocate marks according to those criteria. If your essay *does*
contain the required arguments and points, then you will be awarded
the marks. If it does not, you will not be awarded the marks. This
method is a much more *logical* approach but it does mean that you get
few marks for an original paper. Many tutors may combine both
impression and criterion marking.

Most tutors will probably employ some form of marking scheme
which entails putting some form of grade (A–F) or score (out of 100).
But even these overall scores or grades offer little in the way of detailed
feedback. Others still may use a specific type of grading format which
spells out how the scores are derived and where your particular

strengths and weaknesses lie. Marks are usually awarded in the following areas:

- Introduction
- Development
- Use of literature and research
- Critical awareness
- Conclusion
- Presentation
- References

The development, use of literature and critical awareness are more important than the other areas and so more marks may be available for these areas.

Feedback on your essay

Writing an essay is a very personal thing so getting feedback on your essays may be hard. When you read the tutor's written feedback you may not agree with what he or she has said. Not every tutor will provide you with detailed feedback. You may just get a grade or a mark. If this is so, then you may have to seek out feedback from particular tutors. This can be especially traumatic if the feedback you receive is rather negative. Conversely, if the feedback is wholly positive it will be a real boost to your confidence. In either case, it is important to get feedback on your effort because it will help you to improve your work – correcting particular weaknesses and building on your individual strengths.

The way in which you respond to negative feedback is important. You may feel aggrieved and unmotivated at first, but if the tutor's comments are fair and accurate, then you must begin to use that feedback as part of the process of learning how to write well. Do not be afraid to admit that this section was 'thin' or that you missed out a really important point which was crucial to the essay. You must keep at it and see the whole process as one to which you may take some time to adapt. Try not to be overly concerned with the marks other students get – though this is more easily said than done – and focus instead on your own progress through the course. People learn at their own pace and in their own individual ways. Learning takes time. Concentrate on monitoring your own progress.

Knowledge of results is important for students and a reasonably quick turnaround is essential so that you can work on the feedback you have received on one essay and improve your grade for the next essay. You can expect that your marks should be available about four weeks after the deadline, but do keep in mind that on some courses samples of these essays may have to be sent to external examiners for external moderation. Moreover, if two hundred students submit their essays at the same time, it is not reasonable to expect one specialist lecturer to have all of these marked in four weeks. Tutors and lecturers have an important responsibility and should ensure that you get feedback on your work within a reasonable timescale.

There may be occasions when you feel that the mark you received in the essay is not fair. In such cases you have a right to confront the tutor and state why you feel that your essay warrants a better mark. If you do this, you must be able to offer a reasoned case to support your views and remember that examiners sometimes make errors of judgement, too. Remember also that your essays may be marked by more than one assessor and some essays will be sent to an external examiner from another institution who monitors the standard of work and the fairness of the marking.

Essay checklist

The following are questions to reflect on when writing essays:

- Have I covered all the main issues?
- Is the discussion of sufficient breadth and depth?
- Have I used other people's ideas appropriately and acknowledged these?
- Am I clear about what I have offered as my own ideas and able to offer supportive arguments for these?
- Is the grammar, spelling and punctuation correct?
- Have I got someone else to proofread the essay?
- Is the content of the essay correct and appropriate to answer the question?
- Have I included a complete reference list?

Summary of chapter

In this chapter we looked at the business of writing essays. Be clear about what *sort* of essay you are being asked to write. Then plan, carefully, the body of the essay before you begin to write it. Time spent in planning in this way will be rewarded when you come to hand in your final draft.

6

Doing larger projects

Doing larger projects
These are the things that you must *do:*
<ul><li>Make sure that you understand the aims of the project</li><li>Structure you time</li><li>Work to a timetable</li></ul>
These are the things that you should *do:*
<ul><li>Meet regularly with your supervisor</li><li>Accept constructive criticism</li><li>Present your work in a professional way</li></ul>
These are the things that you could *do:*
<ul><li>Seek out information from unusual sources</li><li>Read a wide range of books and papers – beyond the remit of your study</li><li>Wordprocess and laser print your final report</li></ul>

Aims of the chapter

- To explore types of larger writing projects
- To identify stages in the research process
- To consider preparation and layout of larger projects

As a student, you will be asked to work on longer written projects. Extended essays, case studies, and short research projects are all examples of these. In this chapter, ways of handling larger pieces of work are explored and suggestions made about how to produce a good project.

What is a larger project?

Here are some examples of the sorts of projects that you may have to complete during your training. Clearly, you will not be asked to do *all* of these! Check with the course handbook to find out, in advance, what sorts of projects you will be asked to do.

Extended essay

The sorts of essays that were discussed in the previous chapter were usually of about 1500 words in length. An extended essay may be double this and may even extend to around 5000 words. All of the comments in the last chapter apply here, but also, you need to consider the following: depth of discussion, level of argument used, structure of the overall paper, amount of material that you will draw upon, number of references to other work and to research that you will use. An extended essay is longer than a standard one and allows more room for error. If you have to write a lot of words, the chances of your including shaky arguments or unsupported propositions increases. You need very clear structure in an extended essay which allows your work to unfold in a logical and systematic manner.

Case study

A case study is a descriptive piece that describes the care of one patient in your care. The point needs to be made that a case study should be a *nursing* case study: it should not dwell, in detail, on the *medical* management of the person in question. Also, it is vital that you respect the confidentiality of the person. Use pseudonyms when describing people or places. It is essential that no one reading your work will be able to identify the particular person in question. Case studies are largely descriptive in nature and require even more detailed structuring than is the case with extended essays. Here are some headings to help you to structure yours:

- Introduction to the study
- Short description of the patient
- Short historical account of the patient's medical background
- Reason for admission to hospital or for referral to community nursing service
- Plan of nursing care (physical, psychological, social, spiritual)
- Description of the nursing care that was delivered
- Preparation for discharge
- Evaluation of nursing care given
- Discussion of overall plan of care
- Review of what has been learned from completing the study
- References

Presenting seminars

During your course, you may be asked to present work to your fellow students. The medium for this is usually the seminar. There are at least three educational aims for seminar work: to encourage you to explore a field of study in some depth and to write a paper about it; to share that information with colleagues and to encourage you to develop skills in presenting information to others in a group setting. Typically, you will be asked to prepare a paper prior to the seminar. For the first part of the seminar, you will read or talk through your seminar paper. For the second part, you will discuss your ideas with your colleagues. It is usually best if you do *not* read directly from your work. Instead, prepare a handout with a list of headings that cover the main ideas from your work. Then, supplement these headings with a talk on each of them. This more informal approach encourages group interaction. Most people are easily bored by one person talking for any length of time: the 'handout' approach means that everyone gets a chance to discuss the topic. More details on how to prepare work for a seminar can be found in Chapter 2.

Presenting conference papers

Sometimes, students are asked to contribute to local or national conferences. The standard conference format is that speakers are allocated between half and three quarters of an hour to read a paper. During a further ten to fifteen minutes, the speaker accepts and answers questions from the floor. In terms of delegates, conferences can range from between about 50 and 2000 participants. If you *do* get asked to speak at a conference, take the opportunity. You can gain a great deal of confidence from learning to address a large audience.

In advance, you need to think carefully about how your paper will be structured. For a half hour paper, you will need about 14 pages of double-spaced text. You will be *reading* the text – no one will have the chance to *read* it at the conference. This means that you must pay attention to the *style* of your writing. A conference paper is likely to be more 'conversational' than an extended essay. Also, you cannot, easily, quote references during a conference paper delivery. You need to give your audience advance notice of the issues that you are going to address. Then, you address those issues briefly and clearly. At the end, you summarize what it is you have said. Be wary of packing in too much information too quickly. You need some 'filler' between the main points of your paper in much the same way as a comedian 'chatters' between jokes. The audience needs to know *which* of your statements is an important one. You flag this up by your tone of voice, by stopping to look, directly at the audience and by allowing time, after the statement, for people to think for a few moments. In preparation, then, you first identify your *main* issues. Then you make a rough draft of what it is you plan to say. You try this out on a colleague – not through their reading it but through your reading it *to* them. Having a rehearsal of this sort can quickly help you to decide whether or not you have developed the right style of paper and of delivery.

Also, if you get the chance to go to a conference as a *delegate*, take the opportunity to do so. Conferences offer you the chance to meet other people, to hear what other nurses are doing and thinking about and to reconsider your own ideas about nursing topics. It occurs to both of us that the most important aspects of conferences are *not* what the key speakers have to say but the meetings, discussions and debates *between* the papers. This should also give heart to those who are planning to *speak* at conferences.

Writing for publication

Many students underestimate the quality of their own work. Excellent work should be shared with others. This is how nursing knowledge is disseminated. Many qualified nurses, and teachers in particular, have their work published in nursing journals and magazines. There is no reason why you should not consider your own work for publication.

A published paper is not the same as an essay. The style of a published paper is quite different to that of work submitted as part of a course. First, it is important to read the *Notes for Authors* at the back or front of most journals and magazines. These spell out exactly what the journal or magazine is looking for. You must follow these notes to the letter. It is pointless simply to send in an essay that received high marks. Instead, read the *Notes to Authors*, modify your essay accordingly and then send it to the journal or magazine. Also, make sure that you are familiar with the *style* of the publication that you choose. The *Journal of Advanced Nursing* publishes papers that are very different to those in the *Nursing Standard*. Read copies of both and notice those differences.

Only a small proportion of the material submitted to magazines and journals is accepted for publication. Do not be downhearted if your work is either rejected outright or if you are asked to modify your work substantially. If the former happens, read your work through again, ask a colleague to read it, make any changes that are necessary and then send it off to another journal. If *they* reject it, then you need to reconsider whether or not *this* piece is likely to be published. If, on the other hand, the journal asks you to rework your piece, do exactly what they ask: the editors and reviewers of the journal have considerable experience in these matters. They know, too, what sells the magazine or journal. Follow their instructions to the letter.

Having a paper accepted for publication will enhance your CV and demonstrate that you have something important to say to a wider audience. Do submit work for publication and do keep trying until you have something accepted.

Research projects

The other sort of longer project that you are likely to be asked to produce is a research project. While it is not likely that you will have to undertake a major piece of research unless you do a master's degree, many diploma and degree courses ask that you prepare a dissertation in the final year of the course. Various types of research projects can be identified:

- A literature review
- A short literature review and a research proposal
- A study in which data collected by other researchers is reanalysed

Notes on literature reviewing (project type one)

A literature review is a judgement about the merits or worth of a piece of research. There is no such thing as the perfect piece of research, so all the research that you read may be critically evaluated. The process of doing research has no real end result, it is ongoing and cumulative. It can always be improved upon, refined, expanded and so on. By being critical of other people's research you can learn to discriminate between 'good' and 'bad' research and develop your own ideas about what research you could do. Being a critical thinker is also a very important activity in adult life.

Why is it necessary to be critical of research?

There are several reasons why it is important to be critical of the research reported in journals and books.

- Sometimes researchers get it wrong and make unjustified claims about what can be done or changed on the basis of their results. There may be alternative ways of interpreting findings from a research study which the author may not have thought about. Even researchers have blind spots.
- It can help you to develop your own thinking about a particular area in which you would like to carry out some research.

- As nurses, many of us are guilty of supporting the myth that if something is in print it must be right. This is simply untrue. Researchers are human too. They make mistakes, are subject to bias, and can still manage to have their work published.
- Being critical can lead to new insights into the research domain. A critical analysis of published research promotes creativity in later studies, and can help to uncover key questions which have not yet been addressed.
- You may be surprised to know that most (sensible) researchers are acutely aware of the limitations of their published reports and use this critical awareness to refine their knowledge about the area or the methods they use or the potential practical applications of the research.
- With the growing interest in research and the goal of making nursing a research-based profession, many more nurses are being asked to review critically research findings and to initiate research at ward level. To meet this demand, nurses from all branches of the profession need to be able to read and evaluate critically a particular field of research. This is especially true if you become involved in post-registration courses, undergraduate or postgraduate studies.
- If you are faced with a particular problem on the ward and have to review the research literature, sooner or later you will have to evaluate the research to find out if it will actually help you to solve the problem.
- Research is of little value if it does not in some way influence the practice of nursing. If practising nurses are to implement research findings, then there is a great need for the practitioners and the researchers to work closely together. Practitioners need to be able to evaluate the research professionally if useful dialogue is to be established between these diverse groups.

Positive interaction between the researcher and the practitioner is necessary to avoid the tendency for practical nurses to change practice because something is fashionable or seems like a good idea which might improve patient care. Such an attitude is dangerous and unprofessional.

Essential features of a good literature review

A good literature review has the following characteristics:

- It is objective.
- It is constructive.
- It is unbiased.
- It provides a penetrating analysis.
- It provides a decisive analysis of quality of the research.
- It should be referenced according to established conventions (the Harvard or Vancouver systems. See Chapter 4 for further details).
- It should be organized in a professional way, carefully typed and attention paid to sentence and paragraph construction.

These characteristics should be found in all good literature reviews but unfortunately critical reviews of the literature often lack some of these features. This is due to the fact that evaluating a research report is a very demanding task. However, if you are determined to learn the necessary skills it will pay rich dividends.

Guidelines for evaluating research reports

There are several ways of tackling the problem of evaluating a report. The type of report, the methods used in the study, the area of research and so on, are some aspects which will influence the decision about how to proceed. However, you should try to adopt a questioning approach at each stage of the research as it is reported in the journal to evaluate a piece of research. But the very first questions to ask are of yourself! These are the questions to ask yourself.

- Do I know enough about the research process to understand this *particular* report? If I do not have sufficient knowledge then I have to get that knowledge before an accurate evaluation of the research can be produced.
- Does the report contain technical terms with which I am not familiar? If it does, then I have to do some background reading. Not to prepare in this way is likely to lead to a fairly weak evaluation. A good example here is the use of very specific statistical terms. If you come across new terms like 'mean, mode standard deviation or nominal, ordinal, interval or ratio data' then

you must be willing to find out what these terms mean. Not to do so will result in at best a superficial understanding of the study and an inadequate basis for evaluating it. These questions are essential to our *understanding* of a research report so do not be afraid to ask them.

- Who is the researcher and what is his/her background? A nurse with a background in psychology may approach a problem on the ward differently from a nurse with a background in information technology. Being aware of the researcher's orientation will help you to understand their particular approach and help you to understand any assumptions that the author has made but has not stated in the report.
- Is the problem being investigated clearly stated? Can it be easily researched? Has it been researched already or is the researcher providing a new and creative slant? Does the question relate directly to nursing practice?
- Is the literature reported relevant to the topic? Is the literature review comprehensive or have key references been ignored or missed out? Are the sources current and up to date or has the author relied solely on well known but out of date references? Is the review laid out logically and coherently? Is a summary provided at the end of the review which accurately captures the crucial aspects of the relevant literature and spells out the relevance of this literature for the study?
- Is there a statement about the overall design of the study such as 'case study', 'experiment' or 'survey', which conveys immediately the type of report which is being discussed? Is there a discussion of the relevant theoretical frameworks? If hypotheses are offered are they stated clearly? Is there a straightforward description of what the researcher planned to do and why and how it was done? Would you be able to use the same procedure on the basis of the information provided? Does the researcher define technical terms clearly or does he or she assume these will be understood?
- Is the method used to collect data discussed in sufficient detail? Is a rationale for the choice of method provided? Does it stand up to criticism? What details are provided about the sample used in the study? Was the sample appropriate? Are details about special instruments used in the study such as questionnaires, interview schedules or measuring techniques provided? Is there a discussion of reliability and validity of findings?

- Are the methods used to analyse the data appropriate for the type of data collected? Is the method of data analysis clearly described? Is it easy to follow in a step-by-step fashion? Are the findings presented succinctly with the help of graphs, tables, or highlighted themes? Is there an adequate discussion of the results? Does the discussion emphasize some aspects of the results and ignore others? Is such an emphasis justified?
- Are the conclusions made by the researcher justified on the strength of the findings? Are the conclusions linked closely to the original purpose of the research? Have any new insights been uncovered during the research? Have new research questions emerged unexpectedly from the study? Are the recommendations made by the researcher feasible? Are they excessive and costly? Is a change in nursing practice justified on the strength of these findings or is there a need for more research before embarking on a programme of major change? What are the implications of the study for further research in the field? Does the researcher evaluate the study and point out possible limitations?

Be realistic about your own ability to evaluate research

Of course you will not always be in a position to answer all of these questions straight away. But given time and determination, as you become familiar with a specific area that is of interest to you, your awareness of what has been done and how it has been done will develop quickly. Be patient and try to be aware of your own lack of expertise in certain areas. It is much better to underestimate your own ability to evaluate critically other people's research than to over-estimate it. If you feel unable to answer some of the questions posed above do not worry, it takes time and patience to develop the necessary skills. If you do find it difficult try to discuss some of these questions with a colleague, mentor, a tutor or a research supervisor.

The research proposal (project type two)

Some students will choose to do a shorter literature review and a research proposal. A research proposal is just that: a realistic plan of action for an anticipated research project. The important issue is that such a proposal should be *achievable* if it were to be carried out. The layout of a proposal should be as follows:

- Project title
- Name of researcher
- Name of supervisor
- Department
- Statement of the problem or research field
- Aims and objectives of the project
- Rationale for doing the research
- Brief review of the relevant literature (read the section, above, on reviewing the literature for further details)
- Research design and methods (sampling, data collection methods, validity and reliability; instruments to be used, special equipment needed etc)
- Methods of data analysis (transcript analysis, content analysis, statistical analysis, software requirements etc)
- Ethical considerations (informed consent, ethical committees etc)
- Financial considerations (to the institution, to the individual, stationery, copying, postage, travel etc)
- Other considerations not covered above
- Curriculum vitae of the researcher (see Chapter 11)

Notes on completing a research proposal

A research proposal is a detailed statement of what you intend to do, why you want to do it and how you will go about doing it. It shows your ability to carry through the project and whether the design and methods you have selected are appropriate to the problem you have identified. The process of drawing up a research proposal can help you to clarify your thoughts and methods. It is also necessary to allow other people to examine your project and its methods. This is particularly true of those projects that require clearance from ethical committees.

Writing a research proposal takes a considerable amount of time. You may have to rough out various drafts and the people to whom you submit the proposal may ask you to make changes. Do not be put off by this. Do not refuse to make changes. You run the risk of supervision or support being withdrawn if you do.

Reanalysing existing data (project type three)

Other students may choose to reanalyse data collected by other researchers. Data exist in various formats: as databases on computers, in the form of interview transcripts, in files and records and so on. Before you start your analysis, it is important to draw up a short research proposal, as discussed above. Then, it is important to be very clear about the following issues:

- What *sort* of data are these?
- What sorts of analyses are *appropriate* with these sorts of data?
- What is it that I would like to find out from these data?
- Am I likely to be able to answer my research question from these data?
- Have I the researcher's permission to access these data?
- Am I sure about the criteria for using the methods of analysis that I have chosen?
- Am I clear about how to write up the report that follows the data analysis?
- Will the researcher want a copy of my analysis?

Once the analysis has been conducted, it is important that the findings are written up as a research report. Details of how to do this are contained in many of the references at the end of this book. Make sure that you discuss your plan for the secondary analysis of data with your supervisor before you start your project.

Projects checklist

The following are questions to reflect on when you consider larger projects:

- Am I clear about what I have been asked to do?
- Have I allowed enough time for the project?
- Have I made a sensible and realistic timetable for the project?
- Have I broken the task into a series of sub-goals?
- Have I arranged meetings with my supervisors?

Summary of chapter

Larger projects are like essays, only longer. All the rules of planning and organizing your work apply to these projects. Because they are longer, you have a greater margin for error. Therefore, be very systematic and careful in collating the information you will use, in planning the structure of your project and in working on the final draft.

7

Using computers

Using computers

These are the things that you must *do:*

- Overcome any anxiety you may have about using computers
- Learn the basics first
- Use them regularly

These are the things that you should *do:*

- Learn to use a wordprocessing program
- Buy a 'how-to-do-it' manual that shows you how to use your programs in easy stages
- Go on a computer training course

These are the things that you could *do:*

- Learn to use all the functions in your wordprocessing program
- Write all of your work directly on to the computer
- Use your computer to plan your work and to store your references

Aims of the chapter

- To identify ways in which you can use computers in your study.
- To highlight some of the specific applications of computers.

Why use a computer?

Sooner or later, most students have to learn to use computers. Many people also buy their own. While a few years ago this would have been impossible, the falling prices of computers and their programs no longer make this the case. You may find that your own computer makes a considerable difference to the way you work and the way that you *think* about your work. So why consider buying one? Here are some uses for a personal computer:

- Writing essays and projects
- Keeping notes
- Keeping lists of bibliographical references
- Drawing graphs and charts
- Preparing front covers for folders and projects
- Keeping a diary
- Planning your work
- Managing your finances
- Doing statistics
- Playing games
- Skills for later employment

Most people use computers more for wordprocessing than for any other sort of function. There is real value in using one in this way. Wordprocessing means that you never have to rewrite from scratch. You can put your ideas down in any order you like, play around with them and change your mind. All this before you begin to get down to the real business of writing. The fact that they are so versatile makes them even easier to use than a pad and a pen – once you have learned a few basic functions. That is no overstatement. All you can do with a pad and pen is write, cross out and throw away. The wordprocessor lets you do a lot more than that. Wordprocessing is discussed in a section below. First: what sort of computer should you buy?

What sort of computer?

Two things tend to dictate what computer you buy. The first is money. The second is how you will use the computer. Nowadays, a powerful computer costs a few hundred pounds. Though money is likely to be tight, it is worth considering whether it would be practical to take out a loan to buy one.

The most common computer is the PC or personal computer. This is also known as an 'IBM clone'. IBM set the standard for personal computers in 1981 and all other manufacturers have tended to follow their lead. The personal computer is one that is most versatile.

There are three main elements to a computer. First, there is the main box that holds the central processing unit, the disc drives and the memory. Then there is the keyboard. The monitor contains the screen that you view your work on and the printer is where you get your output. Most computers are not sold with printers and you should include the price of a printer in an estimate that you make when you are looking to buy.

The main box will contain the main computing chip which will drive your computer. Currently, the standard chips are 386s and 486s. The 486 chips run at higher speeds than the 386s and, if you can, it is worth buying the faster machine. Also, you should buy a computer that has a hard disc. A hard disc is like a removable, floppy disc that contains your data except that the hard disc is *not* removable: it remains part of the body of the machine. Hard discs can hold considerably more data than is the case with floppies. Many low budget computers come complete with 40 megabyte hard discs and you can buy them with up to 2 or 3 gigabytes. A 40 megabyte hard disc will hold about 40 times the amount of data that can be stored on a single floppy disc. This may seem like overkill. By the end of your course, though, you will be surprised how much work you have completed and how small a 40 megabyte hard disc can seem.

The keyboard is the most 'subjective' part of the computer. If you are going to live with a computer and if you can type at all, then you should try out a few different keyboards before you make a final decision about your computer. Some people prefer 'clicky' keyboards which feel more like typewriter keys. Other people prefer 'rubbery' ones which are usually softer. If you are going to use one type of keyboard in the college and one at home, it is sometimes possible to match them up by buying from the same source. It makes a surprising difference if you have to keep shifting from one keyboard to another. Also, it is sometimes possible to negotiate a discount in the price if you buy your computer through your college. Many companies offer a special 'educational' price for their computer equipment and software for students.

The third part of the computer is the monitor. Nowadays, these usually have colour screens. Some claim that black and white or 'mono' screens are all you need for wordprocessing. In practice, most people prefer colour screens and the difference in price makes it seem a false economy to buy a mono screen when you could have a coloured one. Most screens are 14" (36 cm), although larger screens are available for special applications.

You have at least three choices when it comes to buying a printer. The cheapest are 'dot matrix' printers which produce output through a series of tiny needle-like projections which hit a carbon ribbon. These are fairly adequate for most basic printing tasks and are available from around £100. Some suppliers will sell them even more cheaply than this and it is worth shopping around. The next stage up is the bubble-jet printer. This produces characters and lines by ink being squeezed through tiny nozzles. Although the principle sounds an unlikely one, the output from these printers is excellent. There is little comparison between a dot matrix and a bubble jet printer in terms of quality. The quality of bubble jet printout is similar to that of a printed page. They also print far more rapidly than dot matrix printers and are almost silent in operation.

The top-of-the-range printer is the laser. These are falling in price all the time and produce the highest quality printout. They remain outside most people's budgets for home use but it is often worth trying to negotiate access to one in your college. Final year projects and dissertations always look a lot better if they are laser printed.

Models

The type of computer described above is called a 'desktop'. While it is not usually particularly large, neither is it very portable. You find a place for it and it usually stays there until you move. You may want to consider two other types of computer: the laptop or the notebook.

The notebook is the most portable computer of all. It is usually about the size of an A4 jumbo pad of paper and weighs around 6 lb (2.7 kg). A notebook has an inferior screen in comparison to a desktop but it usually has a passable keyboard and a hard disc.

The laptop is a larger computer and is about the size of a small briefcase. It is also about twice the weight of a notebook. Notebooks overtake laptops in performance and this means it is possible to buy some very cheap laptop computers if you look around. Also, many companies offer package deals with a laptop, a printer and some software all bundled together. Make sure, though, that the software really is useful. Remember that if a printer does *not* come bundled with your computer, you should buy one. You can plug a notebook or a laptop into a printer in the same way as you can a full-sized desktop.

The advantages of portable computers are obvious. You can carry them around with you and even take notes straight into them (although this is probably not recommended during lectures). However, they are not quite as portable as they seem. Although they are powered by batteries, battery life is still not all that long. You can expect about 3 hours computing between recharges and recharging usually takes about 5–6 hours. You can, of course, work with the machine plugged straight into the mains but this makes it less than completely portable. Also, the weight factor has to be considered. Five or six pounds does not sound very heavy, but it feels it once you have walked round the town with a notebook in your bag.

Buying a computer

Computers are not sold in the same way as other commodities. The best way of buying a computer often turns out to be through the post. The mail order companies offer the most competitive prices, are generally reliable and often offer very good after sales service agreements. It is essential to negotiate an on-site service agreement when you buy a computer. You will not want to repackage the whole thing and send it back if anything goes wrong.

If you buy through the post, you need to know what you want. There are at least two ways of getting to know what you want. First, you can find the local computer expert and let him talk to you about computers. Stop him every few seconds. The computer world, like the nursing and medical worlds, is full of jargon and people who like computers usually like using it. It is essential that you get to know what sort of computer will be right for you. Do not be led to believe that it is essential that you have the latest and fastest machine on the market. The other way to learn about computers is to buy or subscribe to one or more computer magazines. There is now a considerable range of these and most are targeted at the 'business' and the 'home' user. Many of them carry 'buyers' guides' which can be helpful in picking your way through the maze of machinery. Do not be put off by the language. It is not necessary to know how a computer works (from an electronics point of view) and nor is it necessary to learn how to program. Most of us get by with a basic knowledge of how to work with the machine and with an idea of what software is available. Choosing the right software (the programs that you run on the computer) is equally important as buying the right computer. It is sometimes more difficult to know what to buy in the software field. The 'experts' get very fond of their own favourites and use up much energy in trying to convince everyone else that *they* should be using a particular program. This is particularly true in the domain of wordprocessing. The important thing is to try out several programs, if you can, and choose the one that is most likely to suit your needs. Shareware, discussed below, is an excellent way of helping you to do this.

The operating system

All computers need an operating system. MS DOS and DR DOS are the ones most frequently used in personal computers. An operating system works 'behind' your programs and allows your programs to work. They also enable you to do 'housekeeping' tasks such as formatting discs, backing up your hard disc and making copies of floppy discs. You cannot run a personal computer without one and most companies supply an operating system with the computer when you buy it.

A similar but different program is one called Windows. Windows is *not* an operating system but a program that allows you to work with more than one piece of software at once. It also uses graphics (or pictures) to help you move around the program and many consider it to be more user friendly than an operating system used on its own. Not all programs run under Windows but it is rapidly becoming an essential part of computing for many companies and users. You can, however, live without it.

Wordprocessing

The first program you are likely to buy is a wordprocessor. A wordprocessor is the program that will help you to write your essays, type your projects and organize the data in your research project. Here is a list of some of the sorts of features that you can expect to find in a good wordprocessor:

- A cut and paste facility which allows you to move words around your document
- A word counter and spell checker
- A method of drawing lines and boxes
- A method of searching for particular words or phrases and replacing them, if necessary
- A feature that allows you to work with more than one document at a time

Databases

Put simply, a database is any systematic collection of information. If you keep an address book, you own a database. If you store your references on a series of cards, you are keeping a database. Computerized databases are useful for the following reasons. First, they allow you to store huge amounts of information. Second, they enable you to find very specific information, very quickly. Database programs can be useful for storing bibliographic references, lists of names and addresses, for storing other sorts of records and for structuring certain sorts of research data.

Spreadsheets

A spreadsheet offers you a means of working with rows and columns of figures. Anyone who is familiar with working with numbers will know that most collections of numbers can be most easily worked with in the rows and columns format. With a spreadsheet, you can quickly add columns of figures, run simple descriptive statistical tests and generally organize your figure work. If you plan to keep accounts or work with numbers in a research project, a spreadsheet program will prove to be very useful. Examples of commercial database programs include *Quattro* and *PlanPerfect*. Figure 7.1 indicates what a spreadsheet 'screen' looks like.

	A	B	C	D	E
1	34	12	34		
2	45	23	32		
3	34	12	13		
4	56	34	43		
5	65	12	45		

Figure 7.1   Example of a spreadsheet

Shareware

Computer software can be very expensive. It would be a good idea if you could somehow 'try before you buy'. You can with shareware.

Shareware is quite different to commercial software. It has a unique marketing strategy. A shareware program is distributed free of charge (although a charge is usually made for the discs and the handling.) The idea is that you first try the program and then, if you like it, you send away a registration fee to use the program. In the first instance, you usually have between 30 and 90 days to try out the program before you register it. Further, during this time, you are encouraged to make copies of the program for your colleagues and friends. Then, the same principle applies: they are allowed to try out the program and then send off to become registered users if they find it useful.

Advantages

The advantages of the shareware approach are many for the home personal computer user. First, he or she gets a chance to try the program before making a financial commitment to it. Second, the registration fees for shareware are considerably cheaper than buying copies of most commercial programs. Also, the quality of shareware programs is improving all the time and some of the best is easily the equal of commercial software. Finally, shareware offers you the easy approach to learning more about computer programs and to explore a variety of methods of working with data that you may not have been able to if you had to rely on buying commercial packages.

The names and addresses of shareware distributors are available in any of the monthly computer magazines. Such magazines offers include one or two shareware programs on a 'free' disc attached to the front cover. Anyone who is contemplating buying software, or hardware come to that, should read one or two of the monthly computer magazines. There are lots to choose from and all of the bigger newspaper chains carry them.

Not free

Shareware is not free. The idea, as we noted above, is to try out the program, decide if you like it and then pay for it. If you decide not to use the program then you simply give the discs to another person or format the discs for use with other files. The only free programs are those available in the Public Domain. These public domain programs are often distributed by the same people that handle shareware, although it is often not made clear in their catalogues what is shareware and what is public domain.

Computer checklist

The following are questions to reflect on when you use a computer:

- Am I clear about how to start and exit the program I want to use?
- Do I know how to save my work?
- Do I know how to make backups of my work onto floppy discs?
- Have I identified someone in the organization who can help me if I get stuck?

Summary of chapter

This chapter has been all about computers. There is no doubt that personal computing has changed the way we all think about planning and executing written projects. Computers are also vital in research projects and for working on longer projects. Learn to use one and learn to use *all* of the functions that you need. Many people use computers as glorified typewriters. To do this is to miss the point. A personal computer can help you to edit your work in a variety of ways. Use one regularly.

8

Supervision

Supervision
These are the things that you must *do:*   • Make contact with your supervisor early in the course   • Be clear about the things you can and cannot expect from your supervisor   • Meet regularly
These are the things that you should *do:*   • Make good use of the time you spend together   • Keep notes about what happens during your meetings   • Accept feedback from your supervisor
These are the things that you could *do:*   • Be friends as well as colleagues   • Confront difficult issues rather than avoid them   • Seek out feedback from your supervisor, rather than waiting for it

Aims of the chapter

- To examine the nature of supervision.
- To identify what you can expect from a supervisor.
- To learn how to participate in the supervisory process.

What is a supervisor?

Part of the process of becoming a nurse involves other people helping you. One of the most important people in that process is the *supervisor*. You will encounter a variety of sorts of supervisors and here we identify some of the ways in which the term can be used. Generally, though, supervision can be defined as: the process through which one, more senior person, facilitates the growth and development of another colleague, in a professional and educational context. Bearing that definition in mind, it is now possible to consider different sorts of supervisor.

Mentor

Many clinical units and nursing colleges offer a mentorship scheme. This nearly always involves the student's being allocated a senior nurse, for a specified time, who acts as a friend, advisor, role model and resource person. It is important, for both parties, that the student and mentor work well together. It is useful if both sit down together and identify the following:

- The nature and purpose of the relationship
- A timetable of regular meetings
- How they will best get to know each other
- What each requires and expects of the other
- The times each of them will be working. It is important that students work the same shifts as their mentors so far as is possible.
- A backup system of mentoring if the student's mentor is sick, working other shifts or otherwise unavailable.
- Exactly what is expected of the student, given that students have supernumerary status (that is to say that they are *not* an 'official' part of the workforce but are full-time students gaining experience from working in a particular clinical area). Some mentors may need reminding of this fact. Tactful negotiation will help avoid difficulties in this area. It is vital to make sure that the student's role in the clinical area is established clearly and effectively.
- Whether or not assessments are to be a part of the student's stay in the clinical area. There are two issues here. First, the student may or may not be required to be assessed as part of his or her course.

Second, mentors may devise assessment procedures for helping students to evaluate their skill and knowledge levels. Again, it is essential to establish what sorts of assessments will take place *prior* to working in any given area.

The mentor should also be aware of the following:

- Where you are in your educational course.
- What projects and course work you have to complete during the period of mentoring.
- Any particular difficulties that you have experienced up to date.
- Any personal circumstances that may or may not affect your education.

Although mentors are nearly always *allocated* to students, it should be borne in mind that both people in the relationship should be happy to work together. If you or your mentor find that the relationship is not working out, you should, first, talk about the issue and then, if necessary, be prepared to seek a change. You should know whom to approach about changing your mentor should this be necessary. Normally, a teacher in the college of nursing will have special responsibility for organizing the mentorship scheme.

Clinical placements

In this discussion of mentoring and supervision, it is important to think about the *nature* of clinical placements. Project 2000 and other courses encourage students to be given a wide range of experiences in many different sorts of areas in which they may find patients and clients. Traditionally, student nurses were allocated to places in which they looked after sick patients. Thus a 'clinical placement' usually refers to hospital wards and to clinics and people's homes in community settings. The emphasis was on caring for the sick.

Increasingly, the focus of nurses' work has expanded to include monitoring the healthy and advising them on how to stay that way. Therefore, clinical placements may now include: hospital wards, community clinics, well women and well men groups, antenatal clinics, social work agencies, short placements and visits in prisons, schools and residential homes and even visits to health care provisions within large organizations. This expansion of the types of placements that you may get, on the one hand helps to broaden your view of care and of the role of the nurse. On the other, it means that you will need to make sure that you have reliable and regular contact with your mentor or supervisor so that you can make the best of your placement. You are not there simply to *observe* but also to develop a range of personal, interpersonal and practical nursing skills.

Clinical supervisor

Sometimes, the mentor will be clinically based. Your mentor may, for example, be a ward sister or a senior staff nurse. In some colleges, however, mentors are lecturers and you will be allocated a *clinical supervisor* who will help you to work through your clinical learning goals. The clinical supervisor is a person who will observe your clinical performance, help you to practise and learn new clinical skills and who may be responsible for *evaluating* your clinical performance.

Some colleges of nursing will work on a *learning contract* basis. If this is the case, you will be required to sit down with your clinical supervisor to identify new learning goals for that clinical placement. Think carefully about what you want to learn, check with both the college of nursing and with the syllabus what you are *expected* to learn and then meet with the supervisor to draw up the contract. A learning contract will usually contain the following:

- Your name and stage of training
- The goals that you are *required* to achieve while in this particular clinical area.
- The goals that *you* identify for yourself.
- A record of whether or not these goals have been achieved.
- A more general report on your progress through the placement.
- An area to sign to say that you have read the final contract report and, usually, an area in which you can add your own, evaluative comments.

You are normally responsible for making sure that your learning contract is completed. Take your time over the completion of this document and make sure that it is discussed, in detail, with your clinical supervisor. It is an important tool in the learning process.

Other colleges do not use the learning contract but use a much more structured statement of *competencies* that you are required to achieve at key points in your training. Thus, this particular clinical area will have a list of the competencies that can be expected of any student working in that area. These competencies will have been identified by lecturers in the college of nursing and clinical staff working in that area. The competency lists can be used in various ways. They can:

- Act as a checklist for identifying what it is you have to learn in a particular setting
- Help you to monitor your performance
- Be a form of clinical *assessment*
- Form part or all of your final clinical evaluation. In other words, a completed statement of your having achieved a safe level of practice which contributes towards your final grade as a student. You will need to reach certain levels of achievement in order to become a Registered Nurse.

Again, it will be your responsibility to make sure that your statement of competencies is correctly recorded and that the right people get copies of the completed form.

Some colleges combine both the learning contract *and* the statement of competencies. In this case, most of the above points can be adapted to suit the situation. The key things to remember are these:

- The documents are important. They help you to monitor your progress and contribute to your final grade.
- You are responsible for the completion of the documents.
- They are *official* documents and you may not be able to qualify as a registered nurse without them.

Research supervisor

In the final year of your course, you may be required to complete a short piece of research. Completing a research project is a difficult and demanding task. It requires a lot of determination and hard work. The best results are achieved when there is an effective relationship between the student and the supervisor in which the student and the supervisor work *together*. Listed below are some pointers which can help to promote good supervision.

- The ideal situation is to provide a match between the student's research interest and the supervisor's research interests and methodological expertise. In practice this is not always feasible, so the institution should aim to match the student and supervisor at least in terms of the *content area* or the selected *method*.
- To achieve the above, the institution may require that students write an essay on the subject or provide a draft proposal to get some idea of what the student has in mind. These provisional ideas may be assessed and commented on by an internal review panel (team of lecturers in the college) who could make constructive comments and recommendations.
- Another useful approach is for lecturers who have specific projects in mind to *advertise* these projects, in advance of the dissertation year, within the college. Then students who find these projects of interest can discuss them with the appropriate supervisor.

It is useful to be able to discriminate between the roles of the research supervisor and the student. The research supervisor:

- Should provide a *reading list* for the student covering the content area and the methods to be used well in advance of the commencement of the study.
- Needs to allow *adequate time* to meet with the student. One way of ensuring that time is available may be to allocate a particular day or afternoon each week when students can discuss their projects.
- Should insist on *regular written material* from the student which can form the basis of weekly or fortnightly meetings with the supervisor.
- Consider setting a number of aims for the student to achieve before the next meeting.
- Must demonstrate how to make systematic records of background literature.
- Must help the student to select problems and focus his or her thoughts. He or she must stimulate and enthuse students and provide ideas and guidance.

On the other hand, the student:

- Must *plan* the project satisfactorily with the help of the supervisor.
- Ensure that the key problem areas in the research are addressed fully.
- Develop a sound understanding of the background literature.
- Keep accurate and systematic records of what is read.
- Write up the project in small increments as it develops. The value of a good wordprocessing package cannot be understated.
- Remember the supervisor has several other people to direct, so allow enough time for an appointment to be made if problems arise and extra help is needed.

Personal tutor

Many colleges offer a personal tutor system. A personal tutor is usually a lecturer in the college to whom you are allocated at the beginning of your course and whom you stay with throughout that course. The personal tutor is a person who befriends you and who can help with all aspects of your learning and clinical work. The personal tutor may also play a pastoral role and be someone whom you can go to with personal problems. As with mentors, if you do not get on with your personal tutor (or he or she does not get on with you) you are entitled to renegotiate personal tutoring with another lecturer.

You should make use of your personal tutor. Some students go through entire training having never met their tutor. This is a waste of a valuable resource. Make an appointment, early in the course, to meet with your tutor and to set up a series of meetings. Try to make sure that the meetings have a particular focus and that you are both clear on what you expect from one another.

Placement supervisor

A number of your clinical placements will not be in wards or in community nursing situations. During your training, you will also work in a variety of other settings such as children's homes, residential care facilities, schools, education centres, shops, industrial units and

GP practices. During your time in these settings, you may be visited by a *placement supervisor*, usually a member of the college team, who will be responsible for helping you to get the most out of that placement. Talk to the placement supervisor about your aims, your problems and about what you are achieving during your time in the setting. Your placement supervisor is also likely to work closely with other people in the setting and should be able to negotiate extra learning opportunities.

You can also help in the quality control of these sorts of settings. If you can discuss both the pros and cons of your placement, with the placement supervisor, you can help to make sure that other students will gain from the setting.

The purpose of supervision

These are some of the different types of supervisor you will meet. You are unlikely to meet all of them in any given college. Also, different colleges use different labels to describe the people who fulfil these roles.

It is possible to summarize the purpose of *all* types of supervision, as follows. It is the supervisor's task:

- To help you to learn
- To help you to make the most of your learning opportunities
- To ensure that you act in a safe and appropriate manner with patients or clients
- To act as a resource person
- To act as a role model
- To help ensure that you complete projects and course work
- To help you to deal with 'real life' situations in your clinical placements
- To deal with any complaints or difficulties that you may have
- To be a friend and colleague
- To be an occasional counsellor

What can I expect from a supervisor?

It is reasonable to expect certain things from a supervisor. It is the supervisor's task:

- To treat you as a human being
- To meet you regularly
- To give you time
- To offer you support and tuition
- To give you both constructive positive and negative feedback on both your educational and clinical performance
- To be able to represent your interests when your performance is under review

What can a supervisor expect from me?

Your supervisor can reasonably expect things from you. It is the student's task:

- To treat the supervisor as a human being
- To keep appointments and be punctual
- To be prepared to listen to comments that are made
- To be open to advice about both educational and clinical matters
- To be prepared to *self*-evaluate
- To be prepared to work

What happens when it all goes wrong?

Supervision is not an exact science and sometimes it can go wrong. You may find that you do not like the person whom you have been allocated to work with. The supervisor may find that his or her work commitments make it impossible to offer you detailed supervision. Your needs may change. Whatever the reason, it is important that a damaged supervisory relationship is not allowed to continue. What do you do? First and always, you discuss the fact that the relationship is breaking down, with the supervisor. Although this may be painful, it conforms to an important principle: you discuss your grievance with the person involved in that grievance. Also, although the initial confrontation may be painful and embarrassing, it is far less so than the pain and embarrassment that can be caused by *continuing* an unworkable relationship. This sort of situation can lead to your becoming unproductive and can affect both your educational and clinical work.

Sometimes, this sort of open discussion can relieve the situation to the point where you can continue to work together. At other times, you will both agree that a change of supervisor is called for. In this case, you need to approach a more senior person in the college and negotiate a change. It is, of course, possible to make further changes in supervision, but it is probably best to try to make sure that your first change is your *only* change.

Being supervised

So far, we have discussed what a supervisor is and how you might manage the relationship. Another important issue is what you do while in supervision. If the process is to enhance learning, then you need to keep records of what happens when you meet your supervisor. You also need a clear idea of what you want to discuss during your meetings. All of this is helped by the introduction of some *structure*. The following checklist illustrates the thing that you should consider when setting out in a supervisory relationship.

- *Aims and objectives*. Be clear about what you want from the relationship. It helps if you can formulate, as clearly as possible, what the aims and objectives of the relationship are. An aim is a clear but general statement of what you would like to achieve during the supervisory relationship. Objectives are more specific statements of how you will achieve your aim.
- *Do not play games*. Most people learn to 'play the system', fairly early on in their academic and professional careers. They quickly find out what is and what is not expected of them and what other people do and do not like. Try not to play out the game of 'telling your supervisor what he or she wants to hear'. Try to run the relationship in a open and honest way. You will both get much more out of it if you do.
- *Arranging the meetings*. Think ahead. Before you go to meet your supervisor for the first time, have the dates of your off duty, college study days and other important dates mapped out in your diary. Then, when you meet for the first time, try to arrange a series of meetings with your supervisor, that span the next few months. Do not rely on making fresh appointments each time you meet.

- *Recording the meetings.* After you have met your supervisor and after all subsequent meetings, make notes in your diary about any changes or ideas that you have discussed. Be clear about what *you* have to do and what your *supervisor* has agreed to do for you, prior to your next meeting. It is helpful to make these sorts of entries towards the end of each appointment. That way, both you and your supervisor are clear about any arrangements that you have agreed.

- *Evaluating learning.* Between meetings with your supervisor, you are likely to learn a great deal – both in the clinical setting and in the college of nursing. It helps if you keep a note of the learning that you have achieved. Keep notes either in your diary or in a special notebook set aside for the purpose. Use the notes as the basis of further discussions with your supervisor.

- *Evaluating the relationship.* In an ideal relationship, both parties enjoy all aspects of that relationship. Supervisory relationships are ones that are thrust upon you: you do not normally choose your supervisor. This being the case, it seems likely that *some* supervisory relationships will not run smoothly. You may, for example, respect your supervisor to a considerable degree but not *like* him or her. Reciprocal liking is not a necessary condition for a successful supervisory relationship. However, you do not need to write off the partnership merely because you do not like the other person. Try to evaluate objectively the relationship from all angles. Are you learning from your supervisor? Is he or she helping you to gain in knowledge and skills? Does he or she support you in your clinical work? Does he offer you feedback on your performance? If all of these conditions are met, then it is often reasonable to assume that the relationship is 'working'. The converse is also true. You may like your supervisor a great deal but find yourself learning very little from him or her. Try to be as detached and objective as you can. Stand back and ask yourself what are the best and worst aspects of what is happening between you.

- *Considering the long-term view.* When you first start a course, it is common to want to react *immediately* to what is happening. If, for example, you find that you do not like your first clinical placement, you may have a tendency to ask for a transfer. If you are not happy with a lecturer's teaching performance, you may be inclined either to skip his lectures or to complain about them. Try, if possible, to take the longer view. Discuss some of these issues with your supervisor but try not to act too hastily. Too much dramatic change too soon in the course is likely to be disruptive both to you and to your colleagues.

- *Ending the relationship.* All relationships have to end. At some point, you have to part company with your supervisor. As we have seen, above, such parting may be easy. If you have not liked him or her, you may find the leaving easy. On the other hand, if you have survived three or four years together, you are likely to have become quite fond of each other. If you can, discuss the fact that the relationship is ending and prepare yourself for the time when it finishes altogether. If you have been seeing your supervisor in a *counselling* role, then you may want to think about setting up alternative support systems.

Difficult issues

All of the above supposes that things will go well. There may, on occasions, be difficulties with placements, difficulties with relationships or you may even feel that you are witnessing malpractice. What do you do if these things happen?

Here are some options to consider when you are faced with personal or professional problems in practice.

- You can join a professional organization or a union, so that you have proper support during crises as a professional issue is reviewed. The biggest nursing organization and union is the Royal College of Nursing (RCN) and they have special student rates of subscription. They also have a wide range of student facilities including: cheaper holidays and travel insurance, low cost journal subscriptions and discount on certain goods and services.
- You seek advice from senior colleagues or, if you are a union member, from a union official. It is important to try to seek the help of someone who is not involved in the problem that you are trying to resolve.
- You can raise the matter, directly, with the people involved in the incident. If, for example, you felt that a patient was being neglected, you may want to discuss this, directly, with the person

in charge of the ward. However, it is also a good idea to seek support for such an action from your personal tutor. All hospitals and clinical areas have established complaints procedures and it is important that you are fully aware of the ones that apply in the areas in which you work. Not to follow them or to try to short circuit them may lead to lack of resolution of the problem and you may find your own position jeopardized. If in doubt, always seek advice from others.

- You may, of course, choose the easy way out and ignore problems. However, it must be borne in mind that you are bound, by the Code of Professional Conduct, published by the UKCC, to act in a professional manner and to make sure that patients' interests are always safeguarded. This implies that you *must* act if you feel that you are witnessing a situation that is likely to be detrimental to patient care. Such dilemmas are not always easy to resolve. You need to become aware of the *ethics* of care and you need to learn how to be appropriately assertive. The latter issue is discussed in the next chapter of this book.

What are the issues that you might expect professional organizations to help you with? The RCN can advise you on the following:

- Complaints made about you at work
- Legal problems
- Professional insurance issues
- Leaving the nursing profession
- Professional issues such as staff shortages, skill mix etc
- Career advice
- Personal problems via their counselling service CHAT
- Working abroad
- Obtaining copies of reports and literature on nursing
- Advice on maternity leave
- Disputes at work
- Grievances about employment
- Injuries and accidents at work
- Queries about salary
- Work-related health problems
- Information about post-registration courses in nursing
- Pensions schemes and superannuation

Other issues for nurses

This chapter has considered some of the issues surrounding support and problem solving. It has not been exhaustive. There are many other issues that you may or may not have to face up to during your training as a nurse. Read through the following list and try to anticipate which ones are likely to affect *you* and try to add to the list:

- Coping with death and dying in the clinical area
- Working with sick and/or dying children
- Working in very stressful environments such as trauma units and accident and emergency units
- Gossip and rumour
- Unwanted pregnancy
- Conflict between colleagues
- Using drugs
- Developing a sexually transmitted disease
- Developing a drinking problem
- Making mistakes and being told off for making them
- Wanting to get married and trying to reconcile marriage with your financial status and your student role
- Problems at home which affect your work and study

If you can anticipate some of these before you face them, you can develop strategies for coping. Also, you can begin to think about the resources available to help you in these situations and whom you might talk to about them. Finally, these issues may not affect you, directly, but they may happen to a friend or a colleague. Again, you need to think, in advance, about how best you might help him or her. It has often been remarked that although nurses work in a caring profession, they are not necessarily very good at caring for each other. Part of caring for others involves thinking ahead and learning to have a practical approach to problem solving.

Supervision checklist

The following are questions to reflect on when you consider entering into a supervisory relationship:

- What do I want from a supervisor?
- What are the best and worst things about being supervised?
- How well or badly do I respond to feedback about my clinical performance?
- How will I perform as a supervisor, myself?
- If I were to choose the ideal supervisor, what would he or she be like?
- How would my work be affected if I did not have a supervisor?
- How well or badly do I respond to feedback about my educational performance?
- What are other people's supervisors like?
- How could the supervisory system be improved?

Summary of chapter

This chapter has been about all aspects of supervision. Make sure that you are clear who your supervisors are and how they can help you. Participate in the supervisory process to get the best out of it. Supervisors are there to help you and you need to set up a reciprocal relationship with them to get the best out of the relationship.

9

Being assertive

Being assertive
These are the things that you must *do:*   • Learn to be appropriately assertive   • Be clear about what you want from other people   • Listen to other people
These are the things that you should *do:*   • Decide when you will and when you will not be assertive   • As far as possible, remain in control   • Learn to recognize assertiveness in others
These are the things that you could *do:*   • Go on an assertiveness training course   • Read more about assertiveness   • Try out some assertive interventions on your friends

Aims of the chapter

• To identify different sorts of assertion.
• To clarify why assertion can help you.

What is assertion?

Being a student takes its toll. Sometimes the person's *own* needs become subsumed within the demands of the organization or profession. One positive way of coping with stress in organizations and in the caring professions is to become more assertive. Assertiveness is often confused with being aggressive: there are important differences. The assertive person is the one who can state clearly and calmly what he or she wants to say, does not back down in the face of disagreement and is prepared to repeat what he or she has to say, if necessary. Woodcock and Francis (1983) identify the following barriers to assertiveness:

1 *Lack of practice:* you do not test your limits enough and discover whether you can be more assertive
2 *Formative training:* your early training by parents and others diminished your capacity to stand up for yourself
3 *Being unclear:* you do not have clear standards and you are unsure of what you want
4 *Fear of hostility:* you are afraid of anger or negative responses and you want to be considered reasonable
5 *Undervaluing yourself:* you do not feel that you have the right to stand firm and demand correct and fair treatment
6 *Poor presentation:* your self-expression tends to be vague, unimpressive, confusing or emotional.

Given that most health professionals spend much of their time considering the needs of others, it seems likely that many overlook the personal needs identified within Woodcock and Francis' list of barriers to assertiveness. Part of the process of coping with stress is also the process of learning to identify and assert personal needs and wants.

A continuum may be drawn that accounts for a range of types of behaviour ranging from the submissive to the aggressive, with assertive behaviour being the midpoint on such a continuum (Figure 9.1).

Heron (1986) has argued that when we have to confront another person, we tend to feel anxiety at the prospect. As a result of that anxiety we tend either to 'pussyfoot' (and be submissive) or 'sledgehammer' (and be aggressive). Most people, when they are learning how to assert themselves experience anxiety and as a result tend to be

Submissive approach (pussyfooting)	Assertive approach	Aggressive approach (sledgehammering)
The person avoids conflict and confrontation by avoiding the topic in hand	The person is clear, calm and prepared to repeat what he or she has to say	The person is heavy-handed and makes a personal attack of the issue

Figure 9.1 Three possible approaches to confrontation

either submissive or aggressive. Other people handle that anxiety by swinging right the way through the continuum. They start submissively, then develop a sort of confidence and rush into an aggressive attack on the other person. Alternatively, other people deal with their anxiety by starting an encounter very aggressively and quickly back off into submission. The level and calm approach of being assertive takes practice, nerve and confidence.

Consider the following example of Heron's three types:

The pussyfooting approach

1 'There's something I want to talk to you about . . . I don't really know how to put this . . . whatever you do, don't take offence at what I have to say . . .'
2 'I don't expect you will like this but I think it is better that I say it than keep quiet about it . . . on the other hand, perhaps it's better to say nothing.'
3 'I know that you have an awful lot of work and I don't want to add to it. Perhaps I ought to discuss what I have in mind with someone else.'

The sledgehammer approach

1 'What you do annoys me. If you had any feelings at all, you wouldn't get home so late . . . but that's typical of you.'
2 'I give up with you. I bet you don't even know what I'm upset about . . .'

3 'Everybody round here is busy. I don't know why you think you're so special. I want you to take on another caseload.'

The assertive approach

1 'I would prefer it if you could get home a little earlier.'
2 'I'm feeling angry at the moment and I want to discuss our relationship.'
3 'I would like you to consider taking on Mrs Jones and her family.'

Notice, too, in your own behaviour and that of others, that *posture* and 'body language' often have much to do with the degree to which a statement is perceived by others as submissive, aggressive or assertive. These types of postures and body statements may be described using Heron's three approaches, thus:

The pussyfooting approach

- Hunched or rounded shoulders
- Failure to face the other person directly
- Eye contact averted
- Nervous smile
- Fiddling with hands
- Nervous gestures
- Voice low pitched and apologetic

The sledgehammer approach

- Hands on hips or arms folded
- Very direct eye contact
- Angry expression
- Loud voice
- Voice threatening or angry
- Threatening or provocative hand gestures

The assertive approach

- Face to face with the other person
- 'Comfortable' eye contact
- Facial expression that is 'congruent' with what is being said
- Voice clear and calm

What is notable from these descriptions of three different approaches to confrontation is that the pussyfooting and sledgehammer approaches can have *physical* as well as physiological effects. The person who frequently adopts one of these two approaches in her dealings with others will often find that she is both physically and emotionally stressed by the experience. Becoming assertive is a potent method of learning to cope with all aspects of personal stress. It can also help to overcome *organizational* stress in that the assertive person is rather more likely to express her own needs and wants and, therefore, more likely to be heard.

Why be assertive?

First, you do not *have* to be assertive. You can *choose* the point at which you are or are not assertive. Paradoxically, choosing in this way is a type of assertiveness itself!

Second, being assertive and standing up for your rights means that you do not get frustrated by other people walking all over you. If you are not sure of yourself, it is easy to become a doormat. Once you get into the habit of being one, it often takes a bit of courage to climb out of that position and to assert your rights. It takes practice and determination. Sometimes, you have to learn to be assertive *slowly*.

Third, nursing is a demanding profession. In caring for others, it is easy to find that your own needs are swallowed up because you feel that you should constantly 'give' to others. However, you cannot give constantly. You need to be able to express the idea that you want to live your own life, that you sometimes want to be on your own and so on. If you *are* to express these ideas, you will sometimes need to be assertive as part of the process. Other people can be very draining if you let them.

How can I be more assertive?

You do not have to become assertive overnight. Like all other sorts of learning, it is often better to learn assertive behaviour slowly and gradually. Start with situations that you feel are not particularly threatening. For example, you may choose to take something back to a shop or you may say 'no' to a fairly straightforward request. As you appreciate that it *is* possible to assert yourself without other people reacting too violently, you can explore assertiveness in other contexts. You may, for example, practise some of the following situations:

- Giving valid reasons why college work could not be handed in on time
- Telling a close friend that you will not be able to go to a party
- Saying 'no' to someone who is close to you

You can also go on an assertiveness training course. Such courses may be organized in your college of nursing. They will certainly be run by local colleges, universities and as evening classes. On such courses, you will role play situations that you find difficult and learn how to approach them more assertively. You will do this in the supportive company of other people who find assertiveness difficult. The problem, for some people, is plucking up the courage to enrol on such courses! Remember, though, that everyone who attends them does so for similar reasons to yours: usually because they feel that they lack assertiveness and would like to handle a range of situations more effectively. If you need to, enrol: that, of itself, will be an assertive act.

Assertiveness checklist

The following are questions to reflect on when you consider when you want to be assertive:

- Is it appropriate for me to be assertive in this situation?
- Am I clear about what I want and why?
- Will I be prepared to compromise if necessary?

Men and women

The principles of being assertive apply to both men and women. However, it has to be recognized that, given the way society is organized, it may still be easier for men to be assertive than for women. On the other hand, nursing is a largely female profession and men may have to come to terms with *their* role in such a profession. In the past, it was sometimes assumed that men who took up nursing might be gay. Some male students still feel that they have to 'justify' their role as a nurse. This problem may or may not be complicated by the fact that the idea of *caring* is sometimes seen as a 'female' activity.

Such male and female stereotypes are sometimes reinforced by medical and paramedical staff who assume that 'nurses' will be female. Also, the problem may be even greater for male students who *are* gay but who do not want to be stereotyped by others. As we have seen in this chapter, *all* nurses are likely to need to develop their assertiveness skills.

Sexual harassment

One particular domain in which it is important to learn to be assertive is in that of sexual harassment. It can be a difficult problem for women and, increasingly, for men. Finnis and Robbins (1992) define sexual harassment in the following ways:

- Unwanted physical contact such as touching, patting or pinching
- Demands for sexual favours in return for help with the person's career
- Repeated suggestions for social activity outside work, even after it has been made clear such invitations are unwelcome
- Offensive suggestions
- Suggestive remarks, innuendo or lewd comments
- Displays of sexually suggestive pin-ups or calendars
- Leering or eyeing up a person's body
- Derogatory remarks which are gender-related
- Sexual assault
- Offensive comments about appearance or dress that are gender-related
- Sexist or patronizing behaviour

The RCN guidelines define sexual harassment as: 'unwanted, unre-ciprocated and unwelcome behaviour of a sexual nature which is offensive to the person involved' (McMillan, 1992). Finnis and Robbins offer the following suggestions for dealing with sexual harassment on an organizational level:

- Training in dealing with sexual harassment should be made available to a range of staff.
- Training, alone, is not likely to be sufficient. Managers must be aware of how damaging harassment can be to a person's private life.
- Policies must be drawn up to make sure that everyone within an organization is aware of how important the issue of sexual harassment is and that it is totally unacceptable.

All of this raises questions that you may want to ask yourself about the issue of harassment:

- Are you aware of any policy in the hospital you are working in, regarding sexual harassment?
- What would you consider to be sexual harassment?
- Are you prepared to deal with it if it happens to you?
- Can you think of someone whom you could easily talk to about it?
- Are you aware of what your friends think about the subject? If not, you may want to discuss it with them.

To be able to deal with harassment or to be able to prevent it before it happens is an important part of becoming appropriately assertive. No one should treat you like an 'object' and no one has the right to try to insist on your behaving in a particular way if it is against your own wishes. Nor have they the right to touch you if you do not want that to happen.

Nursing students' bill of rights

Part of becoming assertive is knowing what your rights are. The Royal College of Nursing's Association of Nursing Students has compiled a Bill of Rights. It addresses basic issues which are not only fundamental to the well-being and educational needs of every nursing student but are also essential for patients' safety and quality of patient care. The points of the bill of rights are wide ranging and cover many of the aspects of being a student discussed, so far, in this book. The Nursing Students' Bill of Rights, published by the RCN (and reproduced here with permission) is as follows:

1   The nursing student has the right to question educational methods and curriculum content. There should be clearly defined means for student input into educational planning and for evaluation of both clinical and classroom experience.

2   As a nursing student you have the right to say, 'I don't understand'. You should be able to admit freely to confusion or non-understanding and to ask for clarification.

3   As a nursing student you have the right to question and receive an informed answer. Nursing care is often shrouded in myth and ritual. The student nurse has the right to know why care is being given and how it benefits the patient/client.

4   As a nursing student you have the right to practise safely under supervision. Making a mistake does not infer some intrinsic flaw in one's character. Learning sometimes involves making mistakes which should be corrected by a supportive supervisor.

5   As a nursing student you have the right to decline responsibility for situations outside your sphere of practice or competence. Nursing students are just that. Students studying to become nurses. You should not be expected to take on responsibilities of a qualified nurse under any circumstances.

6   As a nursing student you have the right to bring to the attention of the appropriate authority any act of patient abuse or poor standard of care. Students must not fear recrimination but receive support in pursuit of any complaint exposing detrimental or unsafe practice or patient abuse.

7   As a nursing student you have the right to be treated as a responsible adult. Nursing students often feel that they are not always treated as mature and capable individuals.

8   As a nursing student you have the right to express your feelings, opinions and values. Students should be able to identify and articulate their concerns without being labelled or judged unfairly.

9   As a nursing student you have the right to privacy in respect of your private life. Nursing students are expected to uphold public confidence and project exemplary conduct. However, in areas

such as personal health and sickness or conditions attached to living in nursing homes, students are often subjected to intrusions in their private life.

10   As a nursing student you have the right to state your individual needs, independent of the role of the nursing student. Being a nursing student often obscures the needs of the person. You should not have to sublimate your personal needs because you are a student nurse.

Summary of chapter

This chapter has been about assertiveness. Being assertive can help you to be clear in your dealings with other people. You can, of course, choose *not* to be assertive in various situations but this should be a *choice* rather than a situation that you feel you are forced into. If you are a shy person, learning to be assertive can take time. That time is well invested and becoming assertive can help you to make sure that you get the best out of your life as a nursing student.

References

Finnis, S. and Robbins, I. (1992) Tip of the iceberg? *Nursing Times*, **88**, (48), 29–31.

Heron, J. (1986) *The Facilitators' Manual*. Kogan Page, London.

McMillan, I. (1992) Improper conduct. *Nursing Times*, **88**, (48), 27–28.

Woodcock, M. and Francis, D. (1983) *The Unblocked Manager: a Practical Guide for Self-Development*. Gower, Aldershot.

10

Relating and communicating with others

Relating and communicating with others
These are the things that you must *do:*   • Communicate!   • Listen to others   • Socialize   • Consider what sort of relationships you want   • Be aware of the HIV-AIDS issue   • If you are in a sexually active heterosexual relationship, consider methods of contraception
These are the things that you should *do:*   • Learn how to communicate, appropriately, with people in other roles   • Read about verbal and non-verbal communication   • Reflect on your own communication style
These are the things that you could *do:*   • Attend a communication studies course   • Try out different styles of communication   • Watch other people in a variety of social settings and observe their communication styles

Aims of the chapter

- To explore changing roles and relationships.
- To examine how you fit into your student group.
- To consider friendships.
- To consider gay issues.
- To identify things to do when things go wrong.
- To identify ways of preventing the spread of HIV/AIDS.

When you become a nursing student, a lot of other things happen, too. No one who takes on a course of study and training does so in isolation. Any course and any vocational training involves meeting other people and coming to terms with changing roles and relationships. This chapter explores ways in which you can make those changes more smoothly and the sorts of things you can do if things go wrong. It also contains information about being gay and about how to take precautions against the spread of the HIV viruses.

Roles and relationships

When you leave school or college, you are likely to have done so from a point of view of being a relatively 'high status' person. You are likely to have been seen as one of the more mature members of the school or college community. If you have come into nursing from another job or later in life, the same thing applies. You are likely to have worked your way into a position where you are respected, to a greater or lesser degree, by other people. When you start a nursing course, or any other full-time, vocational and educational course, you do so as a beginner. Nursing is notoriously hierarchical. Even though the profession has loosened up in recent years, there are still a number of rungs on the hierarchical ladder. You, for example, will be a student nurse, later you will be a staff nurse, then a sister or charge nurse and then on to being a senior practitioner, an administrator or an educator. Each shift in level involves a certain change of status. Like it or loathe it, this sort of social ordering exists and you have to learn to live with it. How? A short list of ways of working with and making the most of your position in the contemporary order of things includes the following:

- Get to know all you can about the role you are being asked to play. Find out what is and what is not expected of you as a nursing student. Stay within the limits of the role but explore all aspects of it.
- Get to know well, a number of other students. This will enable you all to cope better with the change of role.
- If you do not like certain aspects of the role, seek to change it. If possible, do this as a *group* and not as an individual. Remember that as a group of people with the same status, you and your fellow students can have a considerable amount of power. Organize discussion groups and meetings. Put your case to your managers or your educators as clearly and as articulately as you can. Appeal less to emotions and more to reason. If necessary, review the chapter on assertiveness, in this book.
- Enjoy the role. You are a student and that means that you can enjoy certain freedoms that other people may not have. You may, for example, be more outrageous and more demonstrative as a student than you will be able to be at other times in your life. Also, you will be able to take advantage of cheaper travel by making sure that you get Young Persons Railcards.
- To a reasonable degree, organize your life. Make sure that you not only set aside study time but that you allow plenty of time to do the things that *you* want to do. Review the chapters, in this book, that describe ways of organizing your work and study.
- Learn from others. Exploit, to some degree, the fact that you are a 'learner'. Ask questions. Refuse to take 'no' for an answer or to be palmed off with a less than reasonable explanation. Try to get senior staff to tell you why they do the things that they do.

Racism

Nursing is a cosmopolitan activity. Just as nursing students come from all parts of the globe, so too, do their patients. Also, being born in the UK is not a determinant of a person's skin colour. Racism, both overt and covert remains a problem in this country as in others. Overt racism includes the use of abusive comments or language in the presence of or about a person from a different culture. Covert racism is more subtle and can be detected in jokes, off the cuff comments or in generalizations that are sometimes made about people of a certain race.

The authors have in front of them a research paper that is concerned with measuring 'negro aggression'. This is just one example of racism. On the one hand, the word 'negro' may not be acceptable to everyone and, on the other hand, the idea of investigating 'negro' aggression suggests that there is *likely* to be a difference between levels of aggression between people of different races or different countries. Nursing students need to consider not only the way they cope with other people's racist attitudes and behaviour, but also need to think long and hard about their *own* views about race and colour. In a report published after the Brixton race riots some years ago, Lord Scarman, the chairman of the committee investigating the riots claimed that racial prejudice was *so* ingrained in the personal and social consciousness that *everyone* was probably prejudiced in this way, to some degree or another. It is important to reflect upon the degree to which this applies to you and your work as a nurse.

Making friends

One of the most positive aspects of changing your role is that you meet new people. Most people, it seems, only make one or two really close friends. The philosopher, Kierkegaard, pointed out that most lifetimes are too short to make many more 'real' friends! Reflect, as you read this, how many people *you* would call really close friends. It seems likely that you will only identify a reasonably small number of people.

Some people find making friends easy. Some are socially skilled, easy to talk to and not particularly shy. Others are less fortunate and find the whole business of meeting people difficult. What can you do to make the process of getting on with other people easier? From a review of the psychological literature, and particularly the work on social psychology, the following factors emerge. These factors can help you to make friends and then make sure that you keep the ones that you want.

- *Look friendly.* Someone said to one of the authors that 'people who *look* miserable probably *are*'. This may or may not be true but you are more likely to attract people more if you look cheerful and approachable than if you do not. Smile at people.

- *Get people to talk about themselves.* Most of us like expressing our opinion. You are likely to find that people like you if you allow them to talk about the things that *they* find interesting.
- *Do not automatically compare your experience with the experience of others.* It is tempting to try to 'cap' what another person says with an experience of your own. It is also easy to find yourself constantly saying 'I know what you mean . . . I'm like that myself . . .'. Try to accept that the other person is talking about *his* or *her* experience. You do not need to compete.
- *Learn to listen.* Listening is both an art and a skill. Many of us are so preoccupied with our own situation that we only *half* listen to other people. You can increase the chances of being *seen* to listen by observing the following behaviours:

  - *Look* at the other person, while they are speaking
  - Maintain reasonable eye contact
  - Use non-verbal prompts: nod your head, smile and so on
  - Avoid rehearsing what it is that *you* want to say and give yourself up, totally, to what the other person is saying.

- *Pay attention to detail.* Get to know what other people do and do not like. Respect those differences. Do not expect that everyone else will share your views and learn to tolerate and accept other people's points of view.
- *Respect people's privacy.* Everyone needs time on their own. If someone says that they want some time to themselves, do not assume that they do not like you. Allow them space.
- *Be yourself.* Learn to be 'normal' and ordinary. You do not have to impress people, nor do you have to be something or someone that you are not. This does not mean that you have to be boring or middle of the road but simply that, in the end, you need to be who *you* are and not a replica of someone you admire or would like to be.

As a general rule, relationships and friendships are reciprocal. If you put yourself out to be friendly towards another person, you increase the chance that they will be friendly towards you. While you should not force yourself on other people, you also need to work at relationships. While you cannot expect people to queue up to be a friend of yours, you can do much to seek out friendship.

Also, of course, nursing is about effective relationships. Friendships in 'private' life can serve as useful models for nurse/patient relationships, and vice versa. As you learn to get on with people better as a professional nurse, so there will usually be an improvement in your personal relationships.

Being gay

Many people find that they are looking for relationships, both emotional and sexual with people of the same sex. In a predominantly heterosexual society, being gay can sometimes be difficult. The most commonly quoted estimate (based on a large-scale survey of people's sexual behaviour carried out by Kinsey in the 1950s) is that 10% of the population is gay. That is to say that one in ten people is likely to have had a gay relationship of some sort. And yet many people still find it difficult to come to terms with being gay.

Nor is it always a simple question of being gay or 'straight'. A number of people find that they are attracted to people of both sexes and can have both emotional and physical relationships with them. This does not mean that bisexual people are any more promiscuous than gay or straight people: it is just that they can feel attracted to a range of people. In the end, most people probably identify themselves as predominantly gay or straight but a significant proportion of people also have the 'occasional' gay relationship or they have some gay experiences in adolescence. The range of ways of expressing sexuality as a human being is broad. One homosexual relationship does not necessarily make you gay, nor does being gay automatically rule out the possibility of having heterosexual relationships.

What is far from clear is the degree to which being gay or bisexual is a matter of physiology or of socialization. It used to be strongly argued that 'no one is born gay' and that gayness was a question of learning a certain sexual identity. In recent years there have been studies that have suggested that there may be biochemical differences between straight and gay people. Whatever the case, many gay people acknowledge that their gayness was established very early in life – well before the age of 12 for many people (Dryden, Charles-Edwards and Wolfe, 1989).

Part of the process of coming to terms with being gay or bisexual is the question of whether or not to 'come out'. Coming out is the process of letting other people know that you are gay or bisexual. Like sexuality, itself, coming out is not a black and white process. There are a number of possible degrees and they are:

- Coming out to yourself. Accepting your own sexuality, whatever form it may take. Sadly, many people cannot or do not even acknowledge their sexual feelings to themselves.
- Coming out to close friends, who do not tell other people. Not everyone talks openly about his or her sexual and emotional life. You may *choose* whom you tell about being gay or bisexual.
- Coming out to your parents. This may or may not be difficult for some people and, for some, needs careful timing. You cannot assume that your parents will automatically *want* to know that you are gay or bisexual and you cannot *demand* that they accept what you tell them.
- Coming out to people with whom you work. You may want to ask yourself whether or not they *need* to know. Again, sexual orientation is not the subject of open discussion in every work situation and you may or may not decide to let people you work with know about yourself in this respect.
- Coming out to everyone. The person who has 'fully' come out lives openly as a gay or bisexual person and is not afraid to make his or her sexual identity known to others. For some people, this is a political as well as a personal act. To come out in this way is to make a definite statement about yourself. Some feel that *not* to come out in this way is to belittle your own sexual identity. Others feel that there is little need to declare your sexual identity so openly. The choice, in the end, is yours.

There is absolutely no compulsion for a person to come out. As in all things, you are at liberty to disclose as little or as much about yourself to another person as you feel comfortable doing. If you do decide that coming out is for you, then you may want to talk the idea through with a colleague or friend whom you can trust and who has already been through the process.

If you do come out, you have to be prepared to cope with people's reactions. While numerous people will be supportive of your decision, some may not be. Some people, for whatever reasons, have prejudices about gay people in the way that people have prejudices about any group of people who are different to them. You cannot necessarily hope to influence that prejudice (although you just might) and you cannot always *anticipate* how particular people will react. All of this is particularly true of telling parents. While many parents are supportive when they find out that their son or daughter is gay, not all parents are. You need to make a shrewd decision, based on how well you know them, about what and how much you tell them. Again, you are under no *compulsion* to tell your parents that you are gay or bisexual. In the end, your sexuality is your own affair.

If you do find that you are gay or bisexual, you will want to know where you can meet other people. Finding a partner, as a gay person, may not be so straightforward as it is for a straight person. If you have come out completely, you raise the chances of finding a partner in everyday life, simply because everyone who wants to knows that you are gay or bisexual. In this way, you stand as much chance as other people in finding a like-minded partner.

Many towns have gay pubs, clubs and discos, where you can meet other gay or bisexual people. Most large towns, too, have a Gay Switchboard – a counselling service for gay and bisexual people who will also help you to locate gay facilities in the town in which you live. As with all forms of sexual activity, if your relationships with people become physical, then you need to be fully aware of how to have safe sex. Considerable information is available both for gay and for straight people about how to enjoy an active sex life without putting yourself at risk from the HIV virus. The Terence Higgins Trust, in London, can send you booklets about safe sex if you are at all unsure.

The secret, as in many aspects of life, seems to be to accept yourself as you are. This is often easier said than done. For many years, being gay was seen as something of a psychological disorder. Up until the 1960s and 1970s, psychiatrists claimed to 'treat' gay people in order (presumably) to turn them into straight people. It is now much more widely recognized that being gay is not necessarily something anyone has much choice over. After all, few would argue that straight people *choose* to be heterosexual. Pockets of prejudice do still exist, however, although the nursing profession, as a general rule, has mostly been fairly liberal minded in its approach to the gay scene. On the other hand, it is important not to reinforce popular stereotypes of nurses. In the past, it was sometimes assumed that men in nursing were almost automatically gay because of their taking up the job at all. While some male and some female nurses are gay, no generalizations can be made about the percentage of people in the profession who are gay or straight.

Questions to ask yourself

- Are you clear about your own sexuality and your own sexual orientation?
- If you are gay or bisexual, who else knows about it? How did you arrive at the decision about whom to tell?
- If you are not gay, how do you feel about people who are?
- If you are not gay, what advice would you give to a colleague or friend who is?
- How do you react to openly anti-gay conversation?

When things go wrong

Human relationships are complex. Sometimes they go wrong. We fall out with people. We fall in and out of love. People let us down and so on. Some psychologists and psychiatrists hold the view that psychological difficulties are largely caused by breakdowns in relationships with other people. If you think of the things that cause *you* most distress, it is likely that you will find yourself thinking about:

- Relationships with other people
- Separation from or breakdown in relationships with others
- Lack of contact with others
- Lack of self-confidence and therefore doubts about whether or not other people will like you

Of course, other, very practical problems can occur. It is quite possible to find yourself intensely worried about money, about studying or about accommodation. It is also possible to become concerned about health, weight and so on. While some of these things can be discussed and resolved with friends, personal tutors or with members of your family, some of them cannot.

Fortunately, other people are also the cure for many of our emotional problems. Again, the psychological and social psychology literature helps to identify some of the main ways of sorting our problems:

- Find a person to whom you can *talk* about your difficulties.
- Remain as sociable as possible. Even if you are not feeling particularly like associating yourself with others, try not to cut yourself off and become socially isolated.
- Accept the feelings that you have. It is a fact that all of us are capable of feeling strong emotions – love, hate, anger, depression – at different times. If we can accept rather than fight those feelings, we are more likely to work through them.
- Continue to work. It is sometimes tempting, when we are miserable or distressed, to have a few days off. It is usually better to stick to a routine and to continue to work. The process of working can sometimes enable us to have some respite from thinking about our problems.
- Make sure that you know where to seek professional help if you need it. Find out where the local counsellor works and how you can contact him or her. Remember, too, that there are nearly always telephone helplines that can offer anonymous and skilled help if you need it. Remember, too, that the Samaritan organization does not exist only to help people who are suicidal: you can ring them to talk through *any* sorts of problems and they are committed to offering a totally confidential counselling service.

It is sometimes the case that nurses are not particularly good at looking after themselves or their colleagues. You need to learn, on the one hand, to look after yourself and to monitor your own health and emotional resources. You need, also, to look out for your colleagues and friends. Because nursing involves such a close relationship with other people who are unwell, it is often possible to overlook the fact that friends and colleagues are also suffering. Just as you would want other people to notice if *you* were suffering, make sure that you keep an eye on other people. This is not to suggest that you should develop a morbid fascination with other people's health, but just that being involved in a caring profession should also mean being involved in the care of colleagues as well as clients and patients.

Safe sex AIDS prevention

No one can be unaware of the urgency of the AIDS issue. Anyone entering into a sexual relationship with another person must be aware of how to prevent the spread of the HIV viruses. The viruses are very fragile and not easily transmitted. They can, however, be transmitted in the following three ways:

- Through unprotected vaginal or anal intercourse
- By infected blood entering the blood stream
- From a woman with HIV to her baby either during pregnancy or during delivery

HIV cannot be transmitted through:

- Coughing
- Sneezing
- Sharing a toilet seat
- Sharing a drinking fountain
- Mosquitoes and other insects
- Eating food prepared by someone who has HIV
- Showers and swimming pools
- Sweat, tears and saliva
- Animals and pets

Straight or gay, it is vital that you practise safe sex if you are having any sort of sexual relationship with another person. Safe sex (or 'safer sex' as it is sometimes referred to) involves adopting safer sexual activities and excluding those that have a higher risk for the transmission of the HIV viruses. Safe sex is described, in detail, in publications supplied by the Terence Higgins Trust and which are referred to below. Essentially, safer sex is any kind of sex which reduces or eliminates the risk of body fluids getting from one person into the other's body. Some examples of safer sex are hugging, kissing and masturbation. Penetrative sex is more risky as are a number of other forms of direct sexual contact.

Using condoms in all forms of straight and gay sex can reduce the risk of HIV infection and it is important to learn how to use them properly.

Controlling the spread of HIV infection

As a student nurse, you are likely to come into contact with people who have HIV infection or AIDS and it is important to take precautions to prevent spread. The following are simple guidelines, recommended by the Terence Higgins Trust but you *must* consult your hospital's own guidelines regarding contact with people who have AIDS or are HIV positive.

- Spilt blood and other body fluids should be cleaned up with household bleach diluted one part in ten parts of water. Rubber gloves should be worn.
- Blood and other body fluids in contact with the skin should be washed off with soap and water. Do not use bleach on the skin.
- Cuts and grazes on the skin should be covered with a waterproof dressing until a scab forms.
- Be careful with sharp objects that could carry blood or other body fluids in case they puncture the skin.
- Clothing and sheets soiled with blood and other body fluids should be washed in a machine at a high temperature setting. Rubber gloves should be worn when handling soiled articles.
- Do not share razors and toothbrushes with a person who is HIV positive or has AIDS.
- Crockery and eating utensils should be washed in hot water and detergent.

The World Health Organisation suggests special conditions under which nurses should take particular care in their work. These are:

- Nurses with open skin lesions should cover the lesion with an occlusive dressing or gloves to prevent direct exposure to blood and other body fluids. To protect patients, nurses who have draining skin lesions should not take part in direct patient care and should not handle equipment for patient care.
- Nurses providing HIV-infected persons with home care are at the same low risk of infection as nurses in hospitals and other health care settings. Most infected persons who do not need hospitalization can safely be cared for at home. The precautions outlined above should be observed.

- Since HIV infection in pregnant nurses carries the additional risk of subsequent perinatal transmission, pregnant nurses should strictly observe the precautions.
- In general, an HIV-infected nurse does not pose a risk to patients and restrictions in work are not needed.
- An infected nurse's personal doctor should advise on precautions and/or restrictions to protect patients on whether the patients pose a risk to the nurse and, if so, suggest changes in work assignment (WHO, 1988).

Finally, all nurses need to be aware of the *universal precautions* which should be followed *for all patients, all the time*, regardless of what is or is not known about their levels of risk or their serological status. Pratt (1991) identifies the precautions as follows:

- Operating department nurses must routinely use appropriate barrier precautions to prevent skin and mucous membrane contact with blood and other body fluids from *all* patients.
- Plastic aprons should be worn under surgical gowns, or gowns used should be made of material that provides an effective barrier against fluid contamination with blood or other body fluids, excretions or secretions.
- Protective eyewear or face shields should be worn for procedures that commonly result in the generation of droplets, splashing of blood or other body fluids, or the generation of bone chips, regardless of whether or not it is known that a patient is infected with HIV.
- If a glove is torn or a needlestick or other injury occurs, the gloves should be removed and a new glove used as promptly as patient safety permits. The needle or instrument involved in the incident should also be removed from the sterile field.
- Nursing managers of operating departments must ensure that staff employed to clean contaminated instruments (from *all* cases) consistently wear protective clothing, i.e. intact, heavy duty rubber gloves, plastic aprons and gowns, and masks and eye protection (or face shield). Eye protection (or face shield) is especially important as the brushing and scrubbing of dirty instruments may cause an aerosol contamination of potentially infected blood or other body fluids.

The source of much of the information in this part of the chapter is a booklet supplied by the Terence Higgins Trust, 52–54 Gray's Inn Road, London, WC1X 8JU. The organization also supplies a range of other useful leaflets on the subjects of safe sex, AIDS and HIV, including:

- HIV: how to protect yourself and others
- Understanding AIDS
- HIV and AIDS: Information for Women
- What can I do about AIDS?
- HIV and AIDS: Information about mothers and children with HIV infection
- HIV and AIDS: Information for lesbians
- Safer sex for gay men
- Services of the Trust
- Reducing the risks: a leaflet for people who use drugs
- AIDS in the family: Information for parents and carers of children

As the situation regarding all aspects of AIDS and HIV is changing all the time, it is vital to keep up to date in this area and you are advised to make sure that your own knowledge is contemporary. Reading new booklets from organizations such as the Terence Higgins Trust can help, as can reading new books on the topic, as they are published. Most college and university libraries carry stocks of new books about AIDS and HIV.

Birth control

Linked to the issue of safe sex and the prevention of the spread of the HIV viruses is the question of birth control. A variety of methods of contraception are available, including:

- The condom (both male and female)
- The cap or diaphragm
- The sponge
- The pill
- Injectable contraception
- The intrauterine device

- Natural methods
- Vasectomy and female sterilization

One of the advantages of the condom is that it is not only a method of preventing pregnancy, but it is also a method of helping to prevent the spread of the HIV viruses. If you use condoms, make sure that they carry a BSI Kitemark and are not past their 'sell by' date. The Family Planning Information Service points out that you can get further information about contraception from the following sources:

- Your own GP
- Another GP of your choice who gives family planning advice to other GPs' patients too
- A family planning clinic
- A Brook Advisory Centre.

Problem solving

Sometimes, it is possible to sort out difficulties by thinking carefully about what is worrying you. Often, people have what has been called 'free floating anxiety': they feel worried about lots of things without being clear what the problem is. At times like this, it is useful to use a problem-solving approach:

- *Defining the problem.* First, try to be as clear as you can about what it is that you are worrying about. Think carefully and try to summarize your immediate problems in *one sentence*. If it helps, imagine that you are telling someone else what your problem is and that you only have one sentence to tell them with. Defining problems makes them manageable.
- *Identifying a range of solutions.* Next, take a sheet of paper and jot down as many solutions to the single-sentence problem as possible. Exclude nothing. Let your ideas be as practical or as impractical as you can. Generating wild solutions often leads to more possible solutions.
- *Choosing a solution.* From your extended list, exclude, at this stage, the *least* likely ones. The more bizarre ones will have served their purpose: they will have encouraged you to think differently about your problem. Once you have cut down your list in this

way, select just *one* solution that seems to fit the problem best.

- *Putting the solution into practice*. This is often the most difficult part. Make a contract with yourself to try out the solution that you have identified. This may take a considerable amount of self-discipline but once you start, you will find the process becoming easier. Give yourself a reasonable amount of time to try out the solution and allow yourself to make some mistakes.
- *Congratulate yourself on solving the problem or choose another solution*. If the solution works, do something to celebrate your success. Treat yourself in some way. If the solution does not work, go back to the 'brainstorming' section, above, and select another solution.

Using a logical and structured way of problem solving will enable you to cope with many practical and emotional problems. The *structure* usually makes things bearable and manageable. Another, reflective, approach to problem solving is through the use of *focusing*. This method was developed by Eugene Gendlin and a version of it is as follows:

1 Sit quietly and breathe deeply for a while. Allow yourself to relax completely. Notice the thoughts and feelings that flood into your mind. Slowly, but without worrying too much, identify each one.
2 Having identified each thought or feeling that comes drifting into your mind, find some way of 'packaging up' each of those thoughts and feelings. Some people find it easiest to imagine actually wrapping each issue up into a parcel. Others imagine putting each item into a box and sealing it with tape. However you do it, allow each thought or feeling to be packaged in some way. Then imagine those thoughts or feelings, in their packages, laid out in front of your. Notice, too, the sense of calmness that goes with having packaged up your thoughts and feelings in this way.
3 Now, in your mind, look around at those packages and notice which one of them is calling for attention. Sometimes there will be more than one but try to focus on the one that is most in need.
4 Now unpack that one particular issue and allow it some breathing space. Do not immediately put a name to it or rush to 'sort it out'. Instead, allow yourself to be immersed in that particular issue.
5 When you have spent some minutes immersing yourself in this way, ask yourself: 'what is the feeling that goes with this issue? Do

not rush to put a label to it: try one or two labels, tentatively at first. Allow the label to 'emerge' out of the issue. This feeling that emerges in this way can be described as the 'felt sense' of the issue or problem.

6   Once you have identified this 'felt sense' in this way, allow yourself to explore it for a while. What other feelings go with it? What other thoughts do you associate with it? And so on.

7   Once you have explored the felt sense in this way, ask yourself: what is the nub of all this? As you ask this, allow the real issue behind all your thoughts to emerge and to surface. Often, the nub or 'bottom line' is a quite different issue to the one that you started out with.

8   When you have identified the nub or the crux of the issue, allow yourself to explore that a little. Then identify what it is you have to do next. Do not do this too hastily. Again, try out a number of solutions before you settle on what has to be done. Do not rush to make up your mind but rather let the next step emerge of its own accord. Once you have identified the next thing that you have to do acknowledge to yourself that this is the end of the activity for the time being.

9   Allow yourself some more deep breaths. Relax quietly and then rouse yourself gently.

Managing stress

Linked to the resolution of problems is the issue of coping with stress. Nursing is a stressful activity. The process of looking after other people, identifying and meeting their needs and facing their discharge or possible death, all takes its toll on the person who does the caring. It is important to develop strategies for managing your own stress level. There are a number of books about coping with stress. Some of the more practical activities that you can use to monitor and lower your stress levels include the following:

- *Maintain a manageable schedule.* Much of the time, nursing involves working different sorts of shifts and frequently changing work and social hours. When you plan your social calendar, make sure that you can *cope* with everything that you plan. Eat properly, exercise regularly and make sure that you get enough sleep.

- *Seek variety.* If you live in a nurses' home or in hospital accommodation, it is easy to fall into a routine of work/sleep/work/sleep. It is also easy to find that the only topic of conversation is nursing. Make sure that you seek out friends who are not nurses and make sure that you get away from the hospital and its staff on a regular basis.
- *Talk to people.* We have discussed this, to some degree, above. If you can cultivate friendships in which you can share your problems and in which you can talk freely about how you feel, you are less likely to bottle up feelings and problems and suffer the physical and psychological consequences of stress.
- *Relax.* There is a wide variety of methods that you can use to help you relax. Here is one simple relaxation script that you can use to help you release tension:

'Lie on your back with your hands by your sides . . . stretch your legs out and have your feet about a foot apart . . . pay attention to your breathing . . . take two or three deep breaths . . . breathe in through the nose . . . and out through the mouth . . . now let your breathing become gentle and relaxed . . . now I want you to become aware of your body . . . starting at the toes . . . try to experience the feeling in your feet and toes . . . try to experience that as though you were inside your feet and toes . . . now become aware of the lower parts of your legs . . . as if from the inside . . . now your knees . . . become aware of your joints . . . become aware of your thighs and the top of your legs . . . experience them as if you were inside them . . . now experience your pelvis and hips . . . now your abdomen . . . as if from the inside . . . put your attention into your chest . . . experience the feeling inside your chest . . . now your hands . . . your lower arms . . . your upper arms . . . imagine being inside your arms . . . now experience your shoulders . . . feel the shoulder joints . . . experience the feeling inside your neck . . . the back of your head . . . now your head itself . . . feel and experience your face . . . the muscles in your face . . . your lips . . . your nose . . . your eyes . . . finally . . . your scalp . . . imagine the feeling as though you were beneath your scalp . . . remaining fully aware of all parts of your body . . . notice which parts you can fully experience . . . and which parts are numb to you . . . see if you can become more aware of those parts of your body . . . now just lie and relax for a few more moments . . . take a couple of deep breaths . . . and slowly . . . in your own time . . . sit up and open your eyes.'

All in all, most of us need to *learn* to relax. Through using simple 'scripts' like the one above, we can teach our bodies and our minds how to slow down and to notice the difference between being stressed and being relaxed.

Counselling

If methods of self-help do not work, you may find yourself seeking out a counsellor. What do counsellors *do*? Some people feel that they are there to give advice, while others think that there is some sort of stigma attached to seeing a counsellor. In fact, neither position is particularly accurate. Most counsellors adopt what has been called a *client-centred* approach to counselling. This means that, rather than giving advice, they help the person to find his or her *own* solutions to the problems. The client-centred approach acknowledges that:

- Given the time and conditions, we can nearly always find our own solutions to our own problems.
- We all live *different* lives. Therefore, it is not usually particularly helpful to offer people advice about how to live *their* lives.
- In the end, we all have to make our own decisions about what we do or do not do. No one can make your mind up for you.
- On the other hand, the process of helping another person to talk through his or her problems can often lead that person to making an important series of decisions about his or her life.

Most counsellors, then, will encourage you to talk, to identify exactly what your problems are and will ask you questions to help you to elaborate. This process of talking things through, in an accepting atmosphere, can be very helpful. Often, the process of being heard by another person is enough. As we hear ourselves talk and as we verbalize the things that are really bothering us, we find the solutions to our problems. It is the bottling up of problems and feelings that cause the difficulty. This bottling up often leads us to confusion about both what the real problems are and what the solutions to those problems are.

Also, there need not be stigma attached to meeting a counsellor. You do not have to be mentally ill or neurotic to see one. In fact people who are mentally ill are more likely to be seen by a *psychotherapist* than a counsellor. Counsellors also know their limits. If they feel that they cannot help, they will refer you on to someone who can.

So, if you want or need to see a counsellor, how do you go about it? You have at least the following options:

- Talk things through with your personal tutor. He or she may or may not be trained as a counsellor and may be able to help you, directly. On the other hand, the policy, in your college may be that personal tutors do *not* act as counsellors. If this is the case, your tutor will be able to advise on how you can get help.
- Many colleges have a student counsellor. Often, they offer a 'walk-in' service and you do not need to make an appointment to see them. Their location is usually described on student notice boards. Alternatively, your personal tutor will know where to find the counsellor.
- You can find the number of various telephone counselling services in the front of the local phone book. Often, too, the telephone numbers are displayed, prominently, on college notice boards.
- If you are a religious person (or even if you are not) you can approach people at your local religious centre. They will either be able to offer you help or they will be able to refer you to people who can.
- You can ask your GP to refer you to a counsellor. Local facilities for counselling vary considerably from area to area and your GP may or may not be able to make an immediate referral.
- You can read about local and national counselling services in college, local and national magazines. Local free papers often carry counsellor phone numbers.
- You can ask trusted friends for advice about whom you might see.
- You can ask the local Citizens' Advice Bureau for the names and addresses of people who can offer you help.

The important thing to appreciate is that there are always people around to help you if you need it. Often, the difficult thing is *asking* for help. Once you have made the first contact with a counsellor, however, that problem is usually resolved fairly quickly. Bear in mind that counsellors are trained to help you relax and to work through your feelings. Also, they are not there to *judge* you in any way.

Communication checklist

The following are questions to reflect on when you consider communicating with others:

- Do I communicate effectively?
- Do other people know what I mean when I communicate?
- What do I do if things go wrong in relationships?
- Do I know how to contact a counsellor if I should need one?

Summary of chapter

This chapter has been about relationships. Communication is an essential part of the nurse's role: learn to be good at it. When things do go wrong, think carefully about how you can resolve problems and, if necessary, seek help from another person.

References

Dryden, W., Charles-Edwards, D. and Wolfe, R. (eds) (1989) *Handbook of Counselling in Britain*. Routledge, London.

Pratt, R. J. (1991) *Aids: A strategy for Nursing Care*. Edward Arnold, London.

WHO (1983) *Guidelines for Nursing Management of People Infected with Human Immunodeficiency Virus (HIV)*. World Health Organisation, Geneva.

11

The future

<table>
<tr><th colspan="1">The future</th></tr>
</table>

These are the things that you must *do:*

- Plan ahead
- Make sure that you are clear about the educational opportunities that exist in your area
- Be clear about whether or not you can be *financed* to complete other courses

These are the things that you should *do:*

- Discuss your future with a senior manager or lecturer
- Be open to moving to other parts of the country or to other countries
- Be organized in your approach to planning your future

These are the things that you could *do:*

- Consider distance learning courses
- Teach yourself
- Undertake further research

Aims of the chapter

- To explore aspects of travel.
- To focus on further study.

- To identify ways of doing well at interviews.
- To consider the future.

Years ago, it used to be thought that education stopped at the end of nurse training. A 'trained nurse' was one who had completed his or her registration course. Today, most nurses work for further qualifications. Also, all nurses need to consider how they apply for jobs and what their plans are for the future. This chapter is about that future. First, though, some points about travel.

Travelling

During and after your training, you are likely to have at least two possibilities of travel: as an overseas placement or as part of an exchange or scholarship. It is always interesting and useful to see how nursing and health care is organized elsewhere and you are well advised to take any travel opportunities that occur. Change in EEC countries has meant that travel in Europe is even easier than before and cheaper flights have encouraged people to travel further. Many hospitals in other countries seek overseas experience for their own students and many will welcome the idea of a student exchange. In the future, various scholarships and funding organizations (such as *ERASMUS*) are likely to be able to help nurses to travel more widely. If you are really keen to travel, try to make sure that an overseas placement is built into the curriculum programme of the college that you are joining.

Preparation

If you can, plan well in advance of your visit. If you are going to countries outside Europe, you may need to be immunized and you must check with your occupational health department what injections you may need. Also, clearly, you need to make sure that your passport is up to date and that you have obtained any visas that you require. Both can involve visits to government departments and both can take time. You may want to consider whether or not you will travel alone or with a friend. Also, you may want to find out whether or not your college offers scholarships or bursaries or whether or not local businesses may be prepared to help you with your funding.

Make sure that you are completely clear about accommodation in the country you are going to. Ask for a letter that confirms the dates of your stay from the organization that is arranging your stay. When you return, do not forget to write and thank everyone who has helped you. Also, consider taking some small, easily packed, presents that you can give to people with whom you stay or who offer you particular help and support. It is often a good idea to take presents that have some connection with the particular part of the UK from which you are travelling. For instance, the authors have found that Welsh 'love spoons' make welcome presents, can easily be wrapped and easily carried at the bottom of a suitcase.

The old rule about packing and money still applies: pack half the clothes that you think you will need and take twice the amount of money you anticipate surviving on. Carry your money as travellers cheques, although you will also need some cash, and credit cards can be useful. Work out the exchange rate before your travel and become familiar with it. In that way, you will quickly be able to work out the cost of things in the country that you are visiting. There is a simple, adjustable currency calculator which is widely available throughout the UK in supermarket chains which helps you to make 'instant conversions' if you find the rate of exchange difficult to work with. Remember that you can only carry on to the aircraft one small piece of luggage. Think carefully about what you are likely to need on the plane: if you decide you are unlikely to need anything, there is no need to have any hand luggage. However, it is often a good idea to take a small toilet bag with you if you are going on a long-haul flight and you are always likely to need plenty of reading material. Do not underestimate the amount of time you may have for reading: you may have to wait at airports and it can help to pass the time if you have a novel or two in your bag. Bear in mind that once you have booked in all your luggage, you will no longer have access to it until you arrive in the other country. If there is a flight-delay, this can mean that some considerable time passes before you see your things again. This is where it can help to pack toiletries and novels in a carry-on bag. Some people make brave attempts to work through textbooks when they travel: light reading is often a better idea. Concentrating on 'heavy' books can be difficult if you are listening out for flight calls or are generally excited.

The night before you travel, make sure that you have packed everything and that you have your passport, your tickets and your money. Make a last minute check of these three items before you leave.

Getting there

If you are flying, you need to arrive at the airport at least an hour before the time of your flight. If you have to travel some distance to the airport, leave yourself plenty of time: there can be numerous delays, from punctures to road works. You may want to consider staying overnight, near the airport, if your flight is an early morning one and you can afford it.

Book in as soon as you arrive at the airport. If you book in early, you are more likely to have a choice about where you sit on the plane. Remember that there tends to be more leg room in the first row of seats and at the emergency exits. You may want to consider the pros and cons of window versus aisle seats. A window seat can give you a better view and gives you a place to rest your head if you want to sleep. On the other hand, you have to climb over someone else if you want to walk up and down the plane. An aisle seat gives you little or no view but offers better access to the toilet and freedom to come and go as you please. The worst seats on planes are usually the middle ones in a row of three.

During most flights, long or short, you are usually 'entertained' fairly frequently. Soon after take-off you are likely to be offered a meal. On longer flights there will be in-flight videos and a whole range of meals and drinks. If you can, avoid drinking alcohol as this tends to be dehydrating. This is sometimes difficult to avoid as it is often packaged with a meal and it takes some people a great deal of self-control to go without. On the other hand, do have frequent drinks of water or soft drinks. Bear in mind that you do not have to take every meal that is offered to you. Although eating on planes can be a diversion, some people find that they are given too much food. Remember, too, that you always have the option of sleeping on longer flights. Indeed, a 'night' is usually created by the cabin crew at some point on the flight: shutters are pulled down over the windows and lights are lowered. Again, you do not have to sleep, but keep it in mind that your fellow passengers may want to. If 'night arrives' and you are in a window seat, try to make sure that you make a visit to the toilet before the person next to you falls asleep.

If you are on a long-haul flight, the pilot will usually keep you informed of time changes as they occur. It is a good idea to keep changing your watch to the current time. This can help you to readjust when you arrive in the country to which you are travelling. It seems to help with jet lag, too. Also, it can help if you can break your journey with short 'stopovers' in other countries as part of your journey. Some travel firms offer very cheap one or two day stays in cities en route to your final destination.

In the country

If you can, allow yourself plenty of time to adjust to your new surroundings. If it is possible, it is a good idea to arrive in a country a day or two before you start working or visiting. Allow yourself some sleeping time, if you need it, but try to adjust to any time changes as quickly as possible. Be prepared for some 'culture shock' even in European countries. Just trying to work out how people order meals in restaurants and how to get service in a bank can take some getting used to. Familiarize yourself with the local transport service: trams and underground trains can often be a cheap and quick way of getting around cities and many offer cheap-rate weekly or monthly passes. Find yourself a local supermarket or shop and thus make sure that you can always buy any basic items during your stay.

If you are in non-European cultures, you may have to make considerable adjustments. If you are going to Muslim countries, for instance, you may have to do a lot of homework about dress and about how to conduct yourself. These issues are extremely important and never assume that, as a visitor, you can somehow 'bypass' local customs. Read as much as you can about the country and the culture before you get there and, if at all possible, talk to someone who has visited the country before.

While you are abroad, it is a good idea to keep a diary of what you do, whom you meet and what you see. It is easy to forget details if you do not jot them down. Also, you may want to keep a list of contact addresses so that you can keep in touch with people. To this end, it is also worth thinking about having some business cards printed before you go. Many supermarkets now have 'do it yourself' business card printing machines that allow you to produce 50 cards cheaply.

Ways of organizing health care and nursing vary considerably in different countries. You are likely to need to spend the first few days adjusting to the changes. Ask questions about the system and, above all *talk*! People want to tell you how they do things and they enjoy it. If you can, avoid making too many comparisons with how things are done 'at home'. Try not to tell everyone that you do things differently in the UK. You may say it once or twice but to keep reminding everyone can become very boring. Do not forget to thank the people that have arranged your visit and/or your stay.

You are likely to find people very hospitable. In many countries, people will invite you to their homes, take you out for meals or make sure that you are looked after at weekends. Do not take such hospitality for granted and when people visit your hospital, try to 'return' some of that hospitality. As a general rule, people in the UK are not particularly good at putting themselves out for visitors.

If at all possible, learn at least the basics of the language of the country which you visit. This may, of course, be impossible, if you are visiting somewhere fairly exotic, but at least learn the words for 'yes', 'no', 'please', 'thank you' and so on. It is usually a good idea, too, to familiarize yourself with place names and with instructions on bus services and underground trains. Although English is widely spoken in different parts of the world, in others French, German or Spanish may be the second language. If you anticipate doing a lot of travelling in your nursing career, it is worth considering learning another language. Knowledge of at least two languages can often help you to get by in others. Whatever your ability or lack of it in languages, it is always a good idea to take a paperback travel guide with you. Some of the best are the *Rough Guides*, which are now available for many non-European countries as well as for all of the European ones. These guides often give you much more detailed and 'local' information than some of the glossier guides. They are also much more useful to students who are likely to be travelling on a strict budget. John Hatt's book about travelling in the tropics is also useful to *all* travellers – not just those who are visiting tropical countries (Hatt, 1993).

Wherever you are travelling to or working, expect some changes of mood. Most travellers, if they are away from their own countries experience mood fluctuations. It is not uncommon, for example, to experience temporary, mild, depression or quite severe homesickness. This can sometimes be helped by simply making a call to someone at home. Otherwise, keep yourself busy during this period and do not be tempted simply to sit in your room and get more fed up.

While you are away, make a point of learning as much as you can about the culture in which you are living. In your free time, explore the town or countryside and try to eat meals in local restaurants and cafés. Remember to record your experiences in your diary. When you return, consider turning some of the content of your diary into an article for one of the weekly nursing journals. Most run short articles written by students and overseas' experience is always topical, although you will not get published *just* because you have been abroad. You need to write, in some detail, about a particular element of your visit or about the local health care facilities.

Overall, enjoy yourself while you are travelling. Try to pace yourself and get plenty of rest. Many people forget that simply taking in new experiences and seeing things done in a different way is very tiring. If you are travelling in the country you have visited, allow even more time for resting. It is easy to overbook yourself and find yourself exhausted. Most people who have travelled themselves, will realize that you want time on your own and time to take it easy. By way of a rough rule of thumb, if you are travelling and visiting different towns and hospitals, allow yourself three days of 'visits' and have the rest of the time free. If you *do* try to fit in too many appointments, you will not benefit from them, anyway: after a while, one hospital will begin to look like another and you will not remember whom you have talked to and whom you have not. Also, do not have too riotous a night life. Allow yourself visits to clubs, discos and restaurants but leave some evenings free as well. In some countries you will have to pay close attention to when and where alcohol can be consumed and, in other countries, alcohol is forbidden. Most countries also have strict laws about the use of drugs and in some, the penalty for possession is death. Also, all the usual rules about relationships and about safe sex apply when travelling – only more so.

When you return from your visit, it is highly likely that you will be required to submit a short report. If you have been given a scholarship, this is likely to be the rule. Prepare the report from the notes in your diary and submit it on time. In that way, the funding body (whether it is your own hospital or a scholarship trust) is more likely to look favourably on your colleagues when they want to travel. Also, consider sharing your experiences with groups of colleagues but do not be tempted to offer elongated slide shows: most people can only look at a few slides of other people's travels. Keep your presentation short and to the point and invite lots of questions.

Further study

Why study further? First, nursing knowledge, like all types of knowledge, is changing all the time. The skills that you have today, will not suffice next year, let alone in five years time. Everyone needs to update. Also, updating is obligatory. The UKCC makes it a condition of continued registration that all nurses undertake regular courses to bring their knowledge and skills up to date. There is, however, more to further study than simply updating. Most people, faced with the challenge of learning new things, find themselves changing as people as a result. Given that we all work in a profession which is linked directly with other people, this focus on personal change is an important one. Just as the people we care for change, so should we, as nurses, change.

Further study is often a necessary part of career development. If you want to become a manager or a nurse educator, it is likely that you will find it necessary to do other courses. Nurse teachers are required to be graduates. If you do not have a degree, you will have to obtain one if you want to teach. If you want to be a manager, a diploma or degree in management is likely to put you at a distinct advantage.

There is a natural hierarchy to further education and training. This ranges from one or two day courses, to doctor of philosophy degrees. Let us consider the rungs on that particular ladder.

- *Short courses and workshops.* Most hospitals and health authorities run short courses 'in house'. Often a nurse teacher is employed to organize short training courses for trained staff and to plan National Board courses of various sorts. The National Board courses tend to offer a certificate of attendance which will be useful as evidence of having kept up to date as part of the UKCC's requirements.
- *Certificate courses.* Colleges, universities and some colleges of nursing offer a variety of certificate courses. Part-time certificate courses usually run over one or two years and full-time courses

over one year. There are certificate courses in management, counselling, teaching and a range of clinically related topics.

- *Diploma courses.* These are usually longer than certificate courses and offer study in greater depth. Like certificate courses, they are offered in a wide range of topics. Just to confuse the issue, some colleges and university departments offer *postgraduate* diplomas which are, strictly speaking, for people who already have a degree. Many institutions, though, allow access to non-graduates who can demonstrate that they have kept up their learning beyond initial nurse training.

- *Bachelor's degree courses.* Increasingly, nursing is being offered as a degree course topic by colleges and university departments. Graduates are usually awarded a Bachelor of Science degree in Nursing or a Bachelor of Nursing degree. Degree courses for those without another nursing qualification usually run over four years. Graduates are normally also entered on the nursing register as a result of completing the course. Often, a shorter degree course is offered for those who are already trained as nurses. Some nursing degree courses are also available as part-time options. Qualifications for entry into degree programmes are usually the same as for any other degree courses. Mature entrants (usually over the age of 21) may be allowed to enter such programmes without the usual 'A' level requirement.

- *Master's degree courses.* There are two sorts of master's degrees: taught degrees and degrees awarded for research. Taught master's degrees are often run on a part-time basis over two or three years. Some colleges and universities offer a one year full-time course. Master's degrees by research involve little or nothing in the way of formal lecturing or teaching. The person who does a master's degree by research works with a supervisor and carries out his or her own research programme. It is essential that a person who registers for a master's degree by research has a clear understanding of the research process. Access to master's degrees in research is possible to those with first (or bachelor's) degrees and, increasingly, to those who can prove that they have the necessary professional and educational experience to be able to complete the course successfully. A number of colleges allow qualified nurses, who have completed diploma courses, to enter their master's programmes. This route is a popular one for those who want to enter the nurse teaching profession.

- *Doctoral degree courses.* In this country, PhD courses are almost always research courses. They do not, normally, have a large 'taught' component – if they have one at all. People studying for a PhD will normally have another degree and will be well versed in research methods. Doing a PhD takes stamina and it is usually completed over a three-to-five-year time span.

Think carefully about what form your further education is to take. You need to consider, at least, the following things:

- Where you hope to work. When you move hospital or job, you need to review what educational opportunities exist in the new area.
- The likelihood of being sponsored. Courses cost money. They also take up time. You need to investigate whether or not your hospital or health authority will pay some money towards your further educational programme. If they do or if they do not, you need, also, to know whether or not they will allow you time off to attend college.
- Where your course will take you. Do not undertake just *any* course. Consider whether or not this particular course takes you nearer to becoming a teacher, a manager or a more highly skilled practitioner. Ask yourself where it would fit in to your longer term career plans. Remember, too, that all the courses that you do should be written into your CV.

Preparing a CV

A CV or curriculum vitae is, literally, your 'life curriculum' or your professional and educational history, on paper. As soon as you complete your nurse training (or even sooner) start to develop one for yourself. A CV will be useful in a number of ways:

- Many employers will ask to see it as part of a job application.
- It will help you to keep an eye on the 'shape' of your career and point you to areas of personal growth and development that need to be calculated.
- If you travel and visit other hospitals and health care facilities, your CV may help you to gain access and will certainly be useful in helping people to review your background and experience.

- You will need to enclose a CV if you are applying for scholarships. Many organizations offer competitive, short and long scholarships which allow nurses to develop research projects or to travel. Often, nurses feel that they could not possibly be awarded such things. Talking to scholarship organizers, however, reveals that many scholarships go unawarded through lack of applicants. If you are interested in a particular research project or in travelling to see health care in other countries, consider, carefully, the idea of applying for a scholarship. Before you do, make sure that you have drawn up a CV.

An example of a CV is given in Figure 11.1. However, you may want to consider what sorts of headings your CV should have. Here are some of the more usual ones:

- Your full name
- Your home address
- Your age
- Your date of birth
- Your nationality
- Your current job
- Your work address
- A record of the schools and colleges that you have attended, with the most recent one quoted first on your list
- A record of your qualifications, with the ones that you have gained most recently at the top
- A list of any courses that you have attended
- A list of your personal achievements, to date
- A short description of what you do in your job
- Your interests away from work
- A list of publications (if this is applicable)
- Other useful information (the fact that you can drive, your computing ability and so on)
- The names and addresses of two referees (if this is applicable and *only* if you have asked their permission first)

Figure 11.1 offers an example of a completed CV. Keep the layout of your CV simple. Type or wordprocess it but do not be tempted to use lots of different typefaces or fonts. Never use a computer graphics package to 'illustrate' your CV. The best CVs are laser printed, in one typeface (or 'font') and stapled together at the top, left hand corner.

Curriculum Vitae

Name: Sally Andrews

Home address: 24 Highgrove Road, Barnesworth, Surrey, SA3 4HT

College address: Samuel Peterson College of Nursing, Paisley Road, Aldershot, Hampshire, HA4 6FN

Date of birth: 18.4.75

Nationality: British

Marital status: Single

Current post: Nursing student

Secondary education:
1986–1993 Bishop Stewart School, Barnesworth, Surrey.

Educational qualifications:
1991 GCSE Passes:

English Language:	Grade A
Mathematics:	Grade A
Biology:	Grade A
Computing:	Grade B
Electronics:	Grade B
History:	Grade B

1993 A Level Passes:

Mathematics:	Grade B
Biology:	Grade B

Courses attended:
An Introduction to the Nursing Process: Petersfield General Hospital, Petersfield, Surrey: 4.4.93

Evaluating Nursing Care: Samuel Peterson College of Nursing, Aldershot, Hampshire: 3.6.93

Work experience:

1990–1992 Paper round, Barnesworth, Surrey.
1990 Work experience: 4 weeks: Bathgate Nursing Home: Avebury Road, Barnesworth, Surrey.

Publication:
Andrews, S. (1993) A student's life, *Nursing Standard*, **3**, 4: 56.

> **Interests:**
> Swimming (Gold medallist. Represented county in National
> Championships: Reading 1992);
> Reading;
> Playing the violin.
>
> **Other achievements:**
> In 1992, I was head girl at the Bishop Stewart School. During the year, I
> helped to develop a new system of student evaluation in which each
> student who left the school received a signed report of their progress
> through the school.

Figure 11.1 Example of a curriculum vitae

Do not be tempted to bind elaborately your CV. As with many things, simplicity is the keynote. Remember, though, that you are trying to sell yourself with your CV. Take your time over putting it together. Before you start, do some brainstorming. A good way to do this is to think back as far as you can into your childhood and then to note down some milestones. Think about your first school. What did you achieve there? Did you win awards for sports or were you made a prefect? Then, move on to your secondary school. Think through each of the years and think about the things you were doing, both inside and outside of school. Make notes, accordingly. Then, move up to date. Make detailed, if rough, notes of the things that you are doing at the moment, the things that you are interested in and the sorts of things you want to do in the future. Once you have brainstormed all of these details, begin to piece them together under the headings, above. Pay particular attention to dates. Make sure that the dates that you quote on your CV are accurate. You do not want to be challenged, at an interview, about the 'missing year' in your CV, especially if its omission was just a mistake. Check your CV carefully for spelling mistakes and then have someone else read it through and comment on it. Have you left anything out? Is the 'style' right? If they did not know you, would they get a good impression of you from your CV? Listen to what the other person says and make adjustments, as necessary.

CVs are dynamic. You need to review and change them fairly frequently. Usually, you will not have to cross anything out. Instead, you will add to it. If you use a computer, it is useful to keep your CV on disc. In this way, you can quickly modify it and even tailor it a little to suit the situation for which you want to use it. A particular job, for example, may call for a slightly different CV to one that you would send in as part of an application for a travel scholarship.

Applying for a job and being interviewed

Like it or not, you will have to face a number of interviews in your career. Some people find the business of *conducting* interviews very traumatic. It is this factor that can help you to overcome your own pre-interview nerves: the interviewers are quite likely to be nervous. You can, however, do much to present yourself in the best possible light at an interview. If you do some work, beforehand, you maximize the chances of the interview, on the day, going well. Also, you should hope to be *fairly* nervous. It has been shown that a certain level of anxiety helps people to achieve their best. If you go to an interview not worrying whether or not you do well, nor whether or not you get the job, you are unlikely to impress anyone at all.

Presenting yourself

There are some fairly simple things that you can do to ensure that you are seen in your best light. These include the following:

- Make sure that the interviewers have what they asked for. Ensure that your application form or introductory letter is complete. If you are asked to present a CV, make sure that it is properly filled out.
- Practise the interview process with a colleague or friend. Ask that person to field you a number of difficult questions and anticipate your answers. Practise answering questions with concise but accurate answers. On the one hand, no interviewer wants you to be monosyllabic, on the other, interviewers tend not to like having to interrupt you so that they can get on with the next question.
- Do your homework. Know something about the organization in which you are being interviewed. If possible, always make an informal (although scheduled) visit, prior to the interview but do not make this visit on the same day as the interview.
- Look your best. It is usually best to dress reasonably formally (but

not flashily) for interviews. It is a mistake to think that people do not notice clothes; should accept you for what you are; or no longer take clothes and appearance into consideration. Spend some time thinking about how you will look but do not spend so much time on it that you fail to relax during the interview. Do not try to stun the interview panel.

- Arrive in plenty of time. You can always stop for coffee near to the interview site. On the other hand, it is not a good plan to leave things too late. It is certainly a bad plan to arrive late. If it is inevitable that you will be late, however, 'phone through to inform the interview panel.

- Prepare some short questions that you can ask when approached by the panel. Do not ask 'impossible' questions ('Could you tell me the history of this unit?'). Keep your questions simple and make sure that they can be answered by the interviewer in a couple of sentences. If you have real anxieties about the job make sure that these are surfaced during your questioning period. Remember, from the discussion, above, that the interview should be a two-way process: you should be finding out about the people who are interviewing you.

Finally, make sure that you really want the job for which you are applying. Perhaps you cannot always make up your mind before you go for interview, but it is a mistake to use interviews merely as 'experience' and to go through an interview process with no intention of taking the job if you are offered it. Remember that many inter-viewers will ask you if you *will* take the job if it is offered you.

The job market and the future

The job market in nursing is never static. As nurses leave their jobs and as others change their careers then vacancies at all levels become available. However, what has happened in the last few years is that the recession has meant that many health authorities have cut their nursing and medical budgets. This has sometimes meant that nurses who have resigned or retired have not, automatically been replaced. Also, the *way* in which care is delivered has changed. Sick people are not necessarily looked after in hospital. Many remain at home and, as health care promotion schemes begin to bite and modern medicine means that the *course* of illness may not be as long as it once was, fewer nurses may be required both in hospitals and in the community. Unfortunately, you cannot assume that you are guaranteed a job when you complete your training. You are likely to have to search for staff nurse jobs in parts of the country other than the one you trained in. You also need to plan ahead and begin to start applying for staff nurse posts well in advance of your final examinations.

You can maximize your chances of securing a post as a newly qualified staff nurse if you follow some of the points covered in this chapter. Make sure that you present yourself, both on paper and in person, as successfully as possible. Invest time in preparing your CV and in practising your interview technique. It is always the case that if there are a number of people applying for a post and all have similar backgrounds and experience, then personal and presentational issues become very important. CVs and interviews do count. Make the most of both of them.

Future checklist

The following are questions to reflect on when you consider your future:

- Am I clear about what I want to do next?
- Have I discussed my career plans with a supervisor or lecturer?
- Have I considered both the personal and professional implications of my next career move?
- What aspects of work do I appreciate most?
- Do I have a detailed CV?

Summary of chapter

This chapter has been about your future. You need to invest time and thought into planning a future career strategy. Time taken in such planning will be rewarded when it comes to applying for jobs and educational courses. As in all things, take a structured approach to planning your future.

We hope that the strategies discussed in this book have proved both interesting and useful. The rest is up to you. Good luck.

Reference

Hatt, J. (1993) *The Tropical Traveller: The Essential Guide to Travel in Hot Countries*, 3rd edn. Penguin, Harmondsworth.

Appendix: UKCC Guide for Students of Nursing and Midwifery*

* Reproduced by kind permission of United Kingdom Central Council for Nursing, Midwifery and Health Visiting

1 Introduction

This guide has been prepared to help the student of nursing or midwifery. It describes the roles of the United Kingdom Central Council for Nursing, Midwifery and Health Visiting (UKCC) and the National Boards for England, Northern Ireland, Scotland and Wales. It is the Council with which students will register once the requirements set out in this paper have been met. The Council has a Code of Professional Conduct, and other guidance and standards papers, concerning professional practice and conduct. The advice set out in this Guide draws on the Council's Code and other policies and this is intended to assist students of nursing and midwifery. Students, will, of course, also receive advice from their educational institutions and, as necessary, the respective National Boards. The UKCC hopes that you will find this information helpful as you embark on an exciting and rewarding career in nursing or midwifery.

2 About the UKCC

The Nurses, Midwives and Health Visitors Acts of 1979 and 1992 established the UKCC and the four National Boards to regulate the nursing, midwifery and health visiting professions. The Council is charged by these Acts of Parliament to establish and improve standards of education and training and professional conduct. The UKCC is the body which governs the professions; it determines the standards for entry to professional education and training and determines the kind, content and standard of education. The UKCC also determines when the right to practise should be removed from an individual. The UKCC's register is the principal means of regulating the professions. The Council's overriding duty is to protect and improve standards of nursing, midwifery and health visiting education and practice in the public interest.

The UKCC's duties can be summarised as follows:

- establishing and improving standards of education and practice;
- maintaining the professional register;
- determining entry requirements for programmes of study leading to admission to the register;
- determining the content, type and length of educational preparation;

- evaluating applications from nurses and midwives qualified overseas who are seeking admission to the register;
- giving advice on professional conduct;
- conducting hearings to determine whether practitioners should be removed from the register because of misconduct or illness which seriously impairs their fitness to practise and
- prosecuting those who falsely claim to be qualified nurses, midwives or health visitors.

3   About the National Boards

There is a National Board for Nursing, Midwifery and Health Visiting in England, Northern Ireland, Scotland and Wales. The National Boards are also established by the same Acts of Parliament and the key role of the Boards is to approve institutions in relation to the provision of courses. In fulfilling this role, the Boards are required to ensure that the courses so approved meet the standards of the UKCC. Each National Board has an important relationship with the UKCC and their respective functions are defined in law.

At the beginning of the educational programme, every student of nursing and midwifery is 'indexed' by the relevant National Board. The Boards will ensure that those entering training meet the Council's entry requirements. When training is completed, the National Boards will confirm to the UKCC that the Council's standards have been satisfactorily achieved and that the individual is therefore eligible for registration with the UKCC. In addition, the director of the educational programme will complete a Declaration of Character form on behalf of the applicant. These two factors – eligibility confirmed by the National Board and good character confirmed by the educational institution – are necessary before the Council will confer registration status and, as a consequence, the legal right to practise and to use the title of 'registered nurse' or 'registered midwife'.

4   The professional register

The UKCC maintains the professional register containing the names of all those who meet the requirements for registration. The register is a single register divided into parts to indicate the type of education completed. The following list indicates the parts of the register:

Part 1   First level nurses trained in general nursing
Part 2   Second level nurses trained in general nursing (England and Wales)
Part 3   First level nurses trained in the nursing of persons suffering from mental illness
Part 4   Second level nurses trained in the nursing of persons suffering from mental illness (England and Wales)
Part 5   First level nurses trained in the nursing of persons suffering from mental handicap
Part 6   Second level nurses trained in the nursing of persons suffering from mental handicap (England and Wales)
Part 7   Second level nurses (Scotland and Northern Ireland)
Part 8   Nurses trained in the nursing of sick children
Part 9   Nurses trained in the nursing of persons suffering from fever
Part 10 Midwives
Part 11 Health Visitors
Part 12 First level nurses trained in adult nursing*
Part 13 First level nurses trained in mental health nursing*
Part 14 First level nurses trained in mental handicap nursing*
Part 15 First level nurses trained in children's nursing*

*'Project 2000' courses

After initial registration, nurses and midwives are required by law to re-effect their registration every three years to be eligible to practise. The requirements to be met for re-effecting registration are determined by the UKCC and may change over time. The UKCC's register is not only an indication of the education which has led to registration, it is also being developed for the recording of additional post-registration qualifications and is a key and central source of information on the professions.

5   The act of registration

Programmes of education leading to registration as a nurse or midwife prepare students for the role and responsibilities of registered nurses and registered midwives. Registration is not simply a bureaucratic process. Registration will confer on you the legal right to practise the profession of nursing or midwifery and to use the title 'Registered Nurse' or 'Registered Midwife'. Registration is an indication that a level of knowledge and skill has been reached and, critically, that patients and clients can be assured of, at least, safe professional care. The act of registration applies equally to doctors and dentists and some other healthcare professionals who have similar regulatory bodies.

6   The position of students of nursing and midwifery

All students will enjoy the same registration status with the Council once the requirements for registration are met, regardless of whether a certificate, diploma or degree programme leading to registration is undertaken. Names will be entered on to different parts of the Council's register, depending upon the programme and field of practice.

7   Advice for all students of nursing and midwifery

The following advice is presented to assist you during your studentship. The Council hopes that this will be of value.

7.1   Clinical experience

All students move through three clearly defined phases of clinical experience:

initially in clinical areas you will observe care being given and, where appropriate, assist registered nurses, midwives and health visitors;

in the next stage you will be a participant observer, where you will be able to help in the giving of care, under the direct supervision of registered practitioners and

finally you will participate fully, in keeping with your level of skill, knowledge and understanding, and under the guidance of registered practitioners.

7.2   Informing patients and clients about your role

All hospital and community staff working in areas where you are present must be aware of the circumstances where you may assist or take responsibility for giving care.

All patients and clients should be informed that you, as a student, may participate in their care as part of your programme of education. They will probably find out first through booklets or leaflets and later, at a suitable time, it will be explained to them personally by the registered nurse or practising midwife who is supervising your experience. Patients and clients must be reassured that you are supervised by a registered nurse, or health visitor, or practising midwife and that this supervision will vary according to the care being given and according to your own knowledge and experience.

Patients and clients should be helped to understand that this supervised practice is an essential element in your education without which you cannot gain your professional experience or qualification.

7.3   Respecting the wishes of patients and clients

Some patients and clients, once they have this information, may not wish you to be present, or participate in their care. This right, which should normally also have been made clear in the written information they have received in advance of admission, must be respected. You must respect the wishes of patients and clients and be particularly sensitive about not remaining when they would prefer you to leave.

7.4   Identifying yourself

You must carry some form of clear identification, giving your name and designation, when working in patient and client areas. You must also introduce yourself accurately both on the telephone and in direct contact with others. Uniform, where worn, must be worn in accordance with the locally agreed policy.

7.5   Accepting responsibility

You will, at times, find yourself in a position where you may not be accompanied by your supervisor or a qualified colleague. You will also experience emergency situations which are naturally alarming. With experience and skill you will become increasingly able and confident to deal with complex and difficult circumstances. As a student, you must not take responsibility for that which you have not been fully prepared or for which you do not feel adequately supervised or assisted to undertake. The UKCC recognises your position and your right to decline, in the interests of patients and clients, to accept responsibility in such circumstances. Any problems of this kind should be raised with your supervisor or teacher as soon as possible.

7.6   Respecting confidence

During your practical placements, you must respect the confidentiality of all information that becomes known to you. Patients and clients have a right to believe and expect that private and personal information, given in confidence, will be used for the purposes for which it was originally given, and not released to others without their consent. Access to patients' and clients' records must be obtained only when required and for the information needed to undertake care. The use of these records must be closely supervised by your supervisor or teacher and you must follow the local policy for the handling and storage of confidential records. You can find further guidance in the UKCC's paper, 'Confidentiality', and this is available on request from your college library or the Distribution Department at the UKCC.

7.7   Making records

From the beginning of your educational programme, you must recognise the importance of accurate, comprehensive and up-to-date records. You should also have a clear understanding of your role in record keeping at all stages during clinical placements. During your studentship, any record that you make relating to the care of a patient or client must be countersigned by the person supervising your educational experience. The Council has produced a separate paper setting out the standards for records and record keeping. As a midwifery student, you must be aware of specific legal requirements relating to midwifery records which can be found in the UKCC papers, the 'Midwives' Rules' and 'A Midwife's Code of Practice'.

7.8   Dealing with complaints

You must be aware of the local procedures for handling patients' and clients' comments, both positive and negative, on the nature of the care received. The person supervising your clinical experience, such as the ward sister or team leader or your teacher, must be contacted without delay if a patient or client indicates to you that they wish to express concern or complain about any aspect of care or service. Any action taken must follow the local complaints procedures. You have a duty to bring any such complaints to the attention of your supervisor or professional in charge without delay.

7.9 Accountability

Accountability is a key element of professional practice. The responsibilities placed on registered nurses and midwives and health visitors are considerable. Professional education and clinical experience equip individuals with the knowledge and skill to exercise discretion and to make judgements and take action. These responsibilities bring to the individual the personal professional accountability for decisions made and action taken. Accountability in practice is a complex matter, as the breadth of practice, the nature and level of responsibility and the very variable circumstances in which care is given, all make differing demands on nurses and midwives. The UKCC has developed issues relating to the exercise of accountability in a separate paper which is available from the UKCC or your college library. In essence, however, the UKCC's Code of Professional Conduct provides the foundation for judgements and action in practice and the Code is explained and set out in Section 9.

8 Nurses, midwives and doctors

Section 5 of this paper described the act of registration and, from that description, it will be seen that the same system exists for doctors when they have successfully completed their training as medical students and are registered as medical practitioners by the General Medical Council (GMC). Doctors and nurses and midwives are key professionals working together in the treatment and care of patients and clients. The relationship with medical practitioners is clearly important and this is reflected, at national level, by the existence of a Joint Liaison Committee between the UKCC and the General Medical Council. Both the UKCC and the GMC have similar expectations of the standards and the conduct of those registered and both Councils make their expectations explicit. The UKCC's Code of Professional Conduct for the Nurse, Midwife and Health Visitor is set out below in Section 9.

9   The Code of Professional Conduct

The Code of Professional Conduct is a statement of the values of the professions and the conduct expected by the UKCC of all registered nurses, midwives and health visitors. The Code places the interest of patients and clients above all other considerations and provides a basis for judgements and actions in professional practice. The Third Edition (1992) of the Code is reproduced in full below.

"Each registered nurse, midwife and health visitor shall act, at all times, in such a manner as to:

- **safeguard and promote the interests of individual patients and clients;**
- **serve the interests of society;**
- **justify public trust and confidence and**
- **uphold and enhance the good standing and reputation of the professions.**

As a registered nurse, midwife or health visitor you are personally accountable for your practice and, in the exercise of your professional accountability, must:

1   act always in such a manner as to promote and safeguard the interests and well-being of patients and clients;

2   ensure that no action or omission on your part, or within your sphere of responsibility, is detrimental to the interests, condition or safety of patients and clients;

3   maintain and improve your professional knowledge and competence;

4   acknowledge any limitations in your knowledge and competence and decline any duties or responsibilities unless able to perform them in a safe and skilled manner;

5   work in an open and co-operative manner with patients, clients and their families, foster their independence and recognise and respect their involvement in the planning and delivery of care;

6   work in a collaborative and co-operative manner with health care professionals and others involved in providing care, and rec-

ognise and respect their particular contributions within the care team;

7 recognise and respect the uniqueness and dignity of each patient and client, and respond to their need for care, irrespective of their ethnic origin, religious beliefs, personal attributes, the nature of their health problems or any other factor;

8 report to an appropriate person or authority, at the earliest possible time, any conscientious objection which may be relevant to your professional practice;

9 avoid any abuse of your privileged relationship with patients and clients and of the privileged access allowed to their person, property, residence or workplace;

10 protect all confidential information concerning patients and clients obtained in the course of professional practice and make disclosures only with consent, where required by the order of a court or where you can justify disclosure in the wider public interest;

11 report to an appropriate person or authority, having regard to the physical, psychological and social effects on patients and clients, any circumstances in the environment of care which could jeopardise standards or practice;

12 report to an appropriate person or authority any circumstances in which safe and appropriate care for patients and clients cannot be provided;

13 report to an appropriate person or authority where it appears that the health or safety of colleagues is at risk, as such circumstances may compromise standards of practice and care;

14 assist professional colleagues, in the context of your own knowledge, experience and sphere of responsibility, to develop their professional competence, and assist others in the care team, including informal carers, to contribute safely and to a degree appropriate to their roles;

15 refuse any gift, favour or hospitality from patients or clients currently in your care which might be interpreted as seeking to exert influence to obtain preferential consideration and

16   ensure that your registration status is not used in the promotion of commercial products or services, declare any financial or other interests in relevant organisations providing such goods or services and ensure that your professional judgement is not influenced by any commercial considerations."

10   Further information

All of the documents referred to in this guide are available from the Distribution Department at the UKCC. Any specific questions and comments should be addressed to the:

Registrar and Chief Executive
UKCC
23 Portland Place
London
W1N 3AF

11   Conclusion

The UKCC hopes that you will find these notes helpful in understanding the key role that you will be fulfilling as a nursing or midwifery student. The UKCC wishes you every success in your programme of preparation for registration and in your career as a registered nurse or midwife.

Bibliography

Adler, R. B., Rosenfield, L. B. and Towne, N. (1983) *Interplay: The Process of Interpersonal Communication*. Holt, Rinehart and Winston, London.

Adler, R. and Rodman, G. (1988) *Understanding Human Communication*, 3rd edn. Holt, Rinehart and Winston, New York.

Alberti, R. E. and Emmons, M. L. (1982) *Your Perfect Right: A Guide to Assertive Living*, 4th edn. Impact Publishers, San Luis, California.

Allan, J. (1989) *How to Develop Your Personal Management Skills*. Kogan Page, London.

American Society of Authors (1983) *The Complete Guide to Writing Non-Fiction*. Writers Digest Books, Cincinnati, Ohio.

Argyle, M. (1983) *The Psychology of Interpersonal Behaviour*, 4th edn. Penguin, Harmondsworth.

Argyle, M. (ed) (1981) *Social Skills and Health*. Methuen, London.

Argyris, C. and Schon, D. (1974) *Theory in Practice: Increasing Professional Effectiveness*. Jossey Bass, San Francisco.

Arnold, E. and Boggs, K. (1989) *Interpersonal Relationships: Professional Communication Skills for Nurses*. Saunders, Philadelphia.

Arnold, M. B. (1984) *Memory and the Brain*. Lawrence Erlbaum Associates, Hillsdale, New Jersey.

Ashworth, P. (1987) Technology and machines – bad masters but good servants. *Intensive Care Nursing*, 3, (1), 1–2.

Baddeley, D. (1983) *Your Memory: A User's Guide*. Penguin, Harmondsworth.

Bailey, R. (1985) *Coping With Stress in Caring*. Blackwell, Oxford.

Balfe, A. (1989) *Master Your Hard Disk*. Sigma, Wilmslow.

Ball, M. J. and Hannah, K. J. (1984) *Using Computers in Nursing*. Reston Publishing, Reston, VA.

Belkin, G. S. (1984) *Getting Published: A Guide for Business People and Other Professionals.* Wiley, New York.

Bond, M. and Kilty, J. (1986) *Practical Methods of Dealing With Stress*, 2nd edn. Human Potential Research Project, University of Surrey, Guildford.

Boone, E. J., Shearon, R. W., White, E. E. *et al.* (1980) *Serving Personal and Community Needs Through Adult Education.* Jossey Bass, San Francisco, California.

Boud, D., Keogh, R. and Walker, M. (1985) *Reflection: Turning Experience into Learning.* Kogan Page, London.

Brookfield, S. D. (1986) *Understanding and Facilitating Adult Learning: A Comprehensive Analysis of Principles and Effective Practices.* Open University Press, Milton Keynes.

Brookfield, S. D. (1987) *Developing Critical Thinkers: Challenging Adults to Explore Alternative Ways of Thinking and Acting.* Open University Press, Milton Keynes.

Broome, A. (1990) *Managing Change.* Macmillan, London.

Claxton, G. (1984) *Live and Learn: An Introduction to the Psychology of Growth and Change in Everyday Life.* Harper and Row, London.

Dickson, A. (1985) *A Woman in Your Own Right: Assertiveness and You.* Quartet Books, London.

Distance Learning Centre (1985) *Stress in Nursing: an open learning study pack.* Distance Learning Centre, South Bank Polytechnic, London.

Edmunds, M. (1983) The nurse preceptor role. *Nurse Practitioner*, 8, (6), 52–53.

Hargie, O., Saunders, C. and Dickson, D. (1981) *Social Skills in Interpersonal Communication*, 2nd edn. Croom Helm, London.

Hargie, O. (ed) (1987) *A Handbook of Communication Skills.* Croom Helm, London.

Harrison, N. (1985) *Writing English: A User's Manual.* Croom Helm, London.

Hawkins, P. and Shohet, R. (1989) *Supervision and the Helping Professions.* Open University Press, Milton Keynes.

Heywood-Jones, I. (1989) *Helping Hands.* Macmillan, London.

Heywood-Jones, I. (1990) *The Nurse's Code: A Practical Approach to the Code of Professional Conduct.* Macmillan, London.

Hill, S. S. and Howlett, H. A. (1988) *Success in Practical Nursing in Personal Vocational Issues*. W. B. Saunders, Philadelphia, PA.

Howard, K. and Sharp, J. A. (1983) *The Management of a Student Research Project*. Gower, Aldershot.

Morton-Cooper, A. (1989) *Returning to Nursing: A Guide for Nurses and Health Visitors*. Macmillan, London.

Murgatroyd, S. and Woolfe, R. (1982) *Coping with Crisis – Understanding and Helping Persons in Need*. Harper and Row, London.

Nelson, M. J. (1989) *Managing Health Professionals*. Chapman and Hall, London.

O'Connor, M. and Woodford, F. P. (1978) *Writing Scientific Papers in English*. Pitman, Oxford.

Scammell, B. (1990) *Communication Skills*. Macmillan, London.

Strunk, W. and White, E. B. (1979) *The Elements of Style*. Macmillan, New York.

The Professional Nurse Developments Series (1990) *Patient Education Plus*. Austen Cornish, London.

The Professional Nurse Developments Series (1990) *Effective Communication*. Austen Cornish, London.

The Professional Nurse Developments Series (1990) *Practice Check*! Austen Cornish, London.

The Professional Nurse Developments Series (1990) *The Staff Nurse's Survival Guide*. Austen Cornish, London.

The Professional Nurse Developments Series (1990) *The Ward Sister's Survival Guide*. Austen Cornish, London.

Turk, C. and Kirkman, J. (1989) *Effective Writing: Improving Scientific, Technical and Business Communication*, 2nd edn. E. and F. N. Spon, London.

Walker, D. (1985) Writing and reflection. In Boud, D., Keogh, R. and Walker, D. (eds.) *Reflection: Turning Experience into Learning*. Kogan Page, London.

Index